Cover Photo Credit: FreeImages.com/Stacy Brumley

21 things

I wish I had known

about

Stuttering

Laurent Lagarde

English translation by Steve Cracknell

www.goodbye-begaiement.com

To Sandrine, Baptiste, Heïdi and Joanna who made me want to progress.

To my parents and to those who have children who stutter; to let you know that there is a happy ending.

CONTENTS

PREFACE BY ALAN BADMINGTON

I feel immensely privileged to have been invited to write this introduction.

Recounting how stuttering impacted so adversely upon his life for so many years, Laurent describes how his efforts to address the issues were thwarted by a dearth of information about the subject. His blog, and subsequently this book, were born out of that frustration and the accompanying feelings of isolation. He was motivated to acquire, and share, relevant material with other interested parties.

Using his own story (as well as leaning upon the experiences of some who have successfully resolved their communication issues), Laurent demonstrates that he possesses an in-depth understanding of the matter by assembling an extensive array of insightful information.

It also incorporates details of the incredibly exciting and transformational journey that he has travelled during recent times. Today, he is "living a wonderful adventure", constantly exploring new horizons and participating widely on the world's stage. Life is now so much FUN!

Laurent's writings (in his native language) have positively influenced the lives of French people for the past seven years. I confidently predict that this translated version will become a much-valued and respected resource for English-speaking persons who stutter (as well as for parents, spouses, partners and professionals).

Reading about the lives of others who have encountered similar issues can provide an interesting insight into how they have dealt (or are dealing) with their respective challenges, as well as offering reciprocal inspiration. It can also alert us to possibilities of which we were previously unaware – allowing us to unearth our true potential when we are willing to expose ourselves to uncertainty and change.

The important and diverse messages that this book conveys will provide encouragement for many people (not just those who stutter) to challenge their restrictive mindsets, so that they may lead more expansive lifestyles. Had such a publication been available when I was younger, I would have been better equipped to deal with my stuttering at a much earlier age.

In common with Laurent, I allowed my fears (and narrow self-image) to inhibit my personal growth for far too long. As a result, my life was, generally, unfulfilled. It took me a long time to realize that there were more rewarding paths available for me to tread. If we retain the status quo, then nothing different is ever likely to happen. Our future will simply be a re-run of the past.

Living a safe and predictable life denies us opportunities to discover just how courageous and extraordinary we are. We gain strength and confidence each time we confront our fears. Unless we place ourselves in more demanding situations, we will remain ignorant of our true capabilities.

Laurent is, indeed, a wonderful role model. I invite you to consider following his shining example by taking steps to free yourself from the gravitational pull of any limiting thinking that may be holding you back. As Laurent (and I) discovered, it can be so liberating! Irrespective of previous disappointments and heartaches, it is never too late to become the person you've always wanted to be.

Well, what are you waiting for?

Alan Badmington

I WISH I HAD KNOWN IT'S POSSIBLE TO

OVERCOME STUTTERING

I started stuttering when I was six. My parents went to see a physician, who said "he'll grow out of it". But I didn't grow out of it. I grew up with it. My mother moved heaven and earth searching for a solution, and so I tried many things: speech therapy, medicines, acupuncture, homeopathy, and more. Once, utterly desperate, she even took me to a healer! I remember a friendly little man with a pot belly wearing a three-piece suit. He swung his pendulum in front of my stomach, placing his hand on my throat to transfer the waves of positive energy. It makes me smile now, but it shows the extent of my parents' hopeless confusion. As a young man, I continued this desperate search, going on a course given by a man who had cured his stuttering, trying sophrology and osteopathy. At that time you were left to your own devices. In the first place, it was difficult to find information on stuttering. Then, when you'd found it, it wasn't always pitched at the right level; often it was intended for professionals.

So I continued with my life, stuttering, letting it dictate my choices: what I ordered in restaurants, my studies, my profession. At work, group discussions were a real ordeal, as was the telephone. I preferred walking along the corridors and talking face-to-face, rather than calling someone on the phone. I developed a real phobia about stuttering. I remember breaking down one day in my boss' office when he asked me to stand in for him and make a speech in public.

By the time I was forty, I thought I would never find a solution; that I would continue to panic whenever I needed to make a phone call, to introduce myself or to speak in public. And then I was saved by the Internet.

Still thinking myself alone, misunderstood and with no hope of a cure, **I suddenly discovered the stories of people who had gone through the same trials and tribulations as I had. And they explained how they had solved their problem!** I was ecstatic. Here were people like me giving me what I needed: information, hope and a user manual. I had discovered a hidden world; I wanted to reveal its existence to French speakers.

So that's what gave me the idea of creating the blog www.goodbye-begaiement.fr in 2009. I wanted to share my experience and above all others' experiences, bring together useful information, and **help other stutterers to save the time I had wasted.**

Originally my aim was to write the kind of blog that I would have wanted to read: a colorful and light-hearted mishmash of constructive stories: I didn't want it to be taken too seriously.

At first, I have to admit, I was a little afraid of the reactions of the french 'VIPs' of the world of stuttering. The only things I had to offer were my sincerity, my own story – which was undoubtedly interesting but not necessarily typical – and the fruits of my documentary research. My surprise at the feedback was as big as my fears had been.

From the beginning my fellow bloggers, Olivier and Alexandre, reacted by sharing my first articles. Daniel, the webmaster of Parole Bégaiement, a French association which gives a voice to those who stutter, also quickly put a link on their site.

Then, I was almost incredulous when I saw eminent specialists such as François Le Huche and Marie Claude Monfrais-Pfauwadel making comments on my articles, fueling my themes and shedding light on the subject with their experience and scientific rigor.

Encouraged by these first reactions, I started looking at Anglophone resources. I made contact with the Stuttering Foundation of America, without great hope that they would be interested in me. I felt like an amateur diver applying to join Jacques Cousteau's team on its next underwater expedition. And there, too, I was surprised. It was the president, Jane Fraser, who kindly replied in person and in French (she has lived in France). She thanked me (thanked me!) for my first translations, and encouraged me to continue by giving me the translation rights for two American bestsellers published by her Foundation. You can't imagine how much that motivated me.

I continued to make contact with numerous former stutterers and therapists who were working together to bring stuttering out of the closet. I shared new teachings and scientific discoveries. Each time, I was welcomed with open arms. These interactions meant a great deal to me.

Since I created the blog, I have read a great deal, discussed, written, and above all passed on the stories of stutterers who have solved their problem. **I have been able to show that solutions exist and, above all, that there are people who have liberated themselves from their stuttering.** This is a long way from the depressing resignation of sayings like: 'once a stutterer always a stutterer' and 'every stutter is unique'.

Yes, stuttering is a complex subject, but through my reading, through all the discussions I have had, and in the translations I have done, **I have discovered there are points which keep coming up again and again. I have also identified what stutterers with positive states of mind and winning attitudes have in common.**

For seven years now, I have been sharing my revelations and enthusiasms on the blog. I have often been asked to write it all down in a book. I am both proud and happy to say that you have that book in front of you. In it, you will find many valuable views and suggestions expressed by numerous stutterers from around the world.

So here you have everything I would have liked to have known at the age of twenty.

Laurent

I WISH I HAD KNOWN THAT STUTTERING IS NOT A FAULT AND IS NOT MY FAULT...

For many years I lived in fear of stuttering.

For many stutterers, Fear is the Black Widow, the Witch Queen, and the Matrix rolled into one. It controls everything. It fuels everything. We are prisoners, unable to escape from the grip of fear's powerful tentacles. We are overwhelmed by it, petrified. It stops us progressing, makes us by-pass the problem, makes us self-centered. It is fear that makes the hidden part of the iceberg of stuttering grow. This metaphor was first used by Joseph Sheehan, an American psychologist who stuttered himself and who has worked a great deal on therapy. The visible behavior patterns of stutterers (repetitions, blockages, word substitution, and the physical effort involved in speaking) represent only the tip of the iceberg. The most important part of the behavioral pattern, the part which maintains the stuttering, is hidden in the depths: fear, shame, the feeling of guilt...

This is demonstrated in the book *Advice to Those Who Stutter*, co-authored by 28 American therapists all of whom have themselves stuttered. In it they share their own experiences and those of many patients. Can you guess how many times the word 'fear' appears in the book? **160.** On almost every page. Which emphasizes how central it is to the subject. Here are two examples of the contributors' reflections:

Margaret Rainey explains:

Every stutterer possesses two very strong and incapacitating feelings in common: Fear and Anxiety. Herein lies the heart of his problem. If the fear of stuttering can be reduced, then certainly stuttering itself can be reduced.

J. David Williams agrees:

Your fear of it is the most disruptive and toughest aspect to deal with. If you weren't afraid of stuttering, you would not have tried so hard and so ineffectively to deny, conceal, and avoid its occurrence. Fear disrupts rational thinking and voluntary motor behavior, including speech. If your fear of stuttering reaches a critical level at any given moment, it becomes literally impossible for you to carry out any voluntary speech modification techniques you have learned, and you'll probably stutter as badly as ever.

Fear isn't the primary cause of stuttering but it maintains and reinforces it. It drags you into a vicious circle, a negative spiral which is difficult to escape. It can be represented like this:

Vicious circle of stuttering

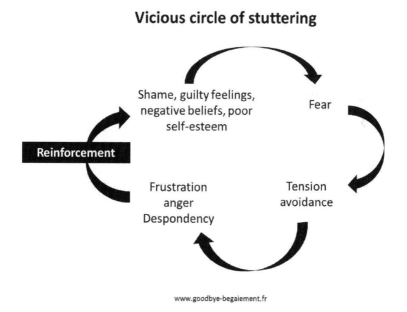

www.goodbye-begaiement.fr

J. David Williams continues:

So an important goal is to learn to keep your fear of stuttering within manageable limits. Try not to give way to blind panic at the approach of a feared speaking situation. You cannot just wish away your old, well-conditioned fear responses, but you can practice overriding the fear. It is always better to go ahead and talk even if you stutter, rather than to remain silent for fear of stuttering. This gives you just a bit more courage the next time!

I can say, without boasting, that this is also my experience. It is the most notable change over the last ten years: **my fear has disappeared**. Or, to be more accurate, the panic has gone. Sometimes I am apprehensive, which is unsurprising, but the terror that haunted me whenever I had to pick up the phone has disappeared. I like to explain this using the plank metaphor which, I think, was conceived by Emile Coué. If you are asked to walk along a plank on the ground, you might well take care to avoid stepping off it but it won't be a problem if you do. On the other hand, if the same plank is placed 300ft above the ground between two buildings you will be much less relaxed and may even refuse to walk it. Even though your legs are still your legs and they can still walk perfectly. That's what happened to me sometimes. Not just sometimes: often. But now I have the impression that the plank is only one foot off the ground and that even if I fall I won't come to much harm.

To summarize, I haven't completely stopped stuttering but I have stopped being afraid. And that changes everything. I would even go so far as to say that it has changed my life.

Stuttering is like a fire fanned by a wind of negative emotions. In order to extinguish the fire, the emotions need to be damped down first. So, at the start of my voyage of discovery I had already made an essential discovery: it wasn't so much that I feared the stuttering in itself, but that I feared it because I **thought stuttering was seriously bad.** In fact, for a very long time, I carried my stutter like a millstone around my neck. I thought of it as a fault for which I was responsible.

I have since realized that this feeling is shared by many people who stutter. As someone who has difficulty speaking, you perceive stuttering as bad, as something to be avoided. It is your fault. You are guilty. You are ashamed of being unable to talk normally and you do everything to hide your stutter. You avoid speaking. You replace one word by another when you are afraid of getting stuck. You pretend to be trying to find the right word or to have forgotten what you intended to say. **Anything is preferable to stuttering. You would prefer people to think that you are incapable of ordinary conversation or that you make grammatical mistakes...**

I was lucky to be working with a psychologist. When I explained that I considered my stutter as a failing she simply replied:

Laurent, stuttering isn't a fault, and it isn't your fault.

For me, those words just clicked. They were a genuine revelation. Understanding that I wasn't responsible made me realize that I had the right to stutter, that I could stutter, and that it was nothing to get worked up about because I wasn't responsible. **The result was that the millstone which was feeding my stutter simply fell off my shoulders.** That simple sentence had pulverized all my negative thoughts, my tension, my avoidance strategies, everything which had contributed to reinforcing my stutter.

Sarah, a young woman affected by stuttering also had the same salutary awakening:

> In the end, I understood that stuttering wasn't a bad thing, as I had thought all those long years. It is simply a part of me. I have blond hair and brown eyes. So what? That's all there is to it. For me, accepting my stutter is to accept myself as I am. I am someone who stutters. For a long while I detested my stutter so I detested myself. **I can honestly say that in working on accepting my stutter, I like myself more and I have more confidence. I feel that I am finally becoming me.**

Here is what **Lee Reeves** has to say on the subject of acceptance. Mr. Reeves is a former president of the National Stuttering Association, the principal American organization in the field.

> Through my own journey with stuttering I have come to believe that acceptance is reaching a state of mind in which we acknowledge both externally AND internally that our inability to speak with the spontaneity and fluidity of others is real but is not our or anyone else's

fault; that while stuttering is part of who we are, it does not define or limit us.

When you relieve yourself of this feeling of guilt you stop being obsessed by stuttering and you can start to advance. You will pass from the stage of 'above all don't stutter' to '**I might stutter but it isn't important. I don't feel guilty especially as I am not doing it deliberately.**'

Note that I am not telling you to accept your stutter without doing anything about it. It is simply that you are not responsible for it and there is no need to be ashamed. It might be genetic, neurological, the result of an accident, etc. But you are not deliberately trying to stutter! It doesn't mean that you are sub-human, or less intelligent, or less competent. This statement has been verified by research and is confirmed by experience every day. All kinds of people stutter, whatever their level of education or profession.

Stuttering doesn't mean you are inferior, simply different. And there is no reason to feel guilty about that difference.

Let's hear what Morgane has to say about that difference. Morgane is Swiss and a member of the Association Parole Bégaiement (Francophone Stuttering Association). In January 2011, she was interviewed by Radio Suisse Romande. It is wonderful to hear her version:

It is the difference which people find a problem, but we are all different, we are all unique. Perhaps I wouldn't be Morgane if I didn't stutter. It's me. Quite simply, my stutter is me! I could almost thank stuttering for being a part of me. I have been able to learn something positive from my bad experiences. Stuttering is a part of me; it is part of my character, my identity.

In *Self Therapy for the Stutterer*, Malcolm Fraser, founder of the Stuttering Foundation of America, cites a therapy participant:

It took me twenty years before I would admit to myself, or anyone, that I stuttered. I didn't want to acknowledge that I was different. Yet that is precisely what I needed to do in order to take the first step toward forging a new and more fulfilling identity.

As the author of *Redefining Stuttering*, John Harrison, says: *"In other words, it is a question of showing yourself as you really are."* Cool, huh?

Of course you may consider that this difference is an imperfection and something to be improved but, as Gary J. Rentschler[1] says:

> Our parents and our friends have imperfections, but we are able to see beyond their flaws and cherish their love and fellowship in spite of their shortcomings. It is our imperfections that make us individual and memorable. **To embrace our flaws is to honor our uniqueness.**

Once you accept this difference without feelings of shame or guilt, a very important transformation will take place in you: **you will agree to talk about it.**

Robert Quesal[2] says:

> An individual who accepts stuttering can talk about it with others. He or she views stuttering as a personal characteristic, similar to height, athletic ability, complexion, sense of humor, reading and writing skills,

---

[1] American therapist who previously stuttered. He is one of the authors of Advice to Those who Stutter.

[2] Idem.

and any other number of things that make us who we are.

I WISH I HAD KNOWN THAT STUTTERING IS JUST ONE PART OF MY PERSONALITY

As Morgane said, stuttering is a part of us; it is a part of our identity... but only a part. We are not stutterers and only stutterers, and that is undoubtedly one of the biggest mistakes we make: we are obsessed by our stuttering to the extent that nothing else gets a look-in. It hides the rest of our unique personal value. Many people prefer to use the term 'person who stutters' rather than 'stutterer' to emphasize that there is more to us than stuttering, that our identity is not limited to that.

I work in a bank. One day I was lucky enough to have an interview with the managing director. Faithful to my resolution to talk about it, I explained to him the impact my stutter had had on my career choices. He replied:

- Laurent, for me your stuttering has never been a problem, even when it was more noticeable than it is now. It is more a problem for you than for other people. More accurately it is not a problem, merely a trait. Your name is Laurent, you have green eyes and you stutter. I even think stuttering can be a strength.

- Woah, hold on there, boss. In two minutes you have summarized something it has taken me 25 years to understand.

- That's why I'm the boss.

To summarize, as it grows, acceptance of your difference will progressively diffuse its benefits throughout your being and transform your relationship with the world. Yes, nothing less! And do you know why? Because, by accepting, you will become reconciled with yourself. By accepting, you will forgive yourself, you will give yourself the love and reassurance necessary for your peace of mind and self-confidence.

When you were angry and in denial, you abandoned yourself to shame, dismay and the rage that stopped you from moving forward and having clear ideas.

"What have I done to deserve this?" "Why do I stutter sometimes and not others?" "Why doesn't it go away?" Denial is the reaction of a child who stamps his feet and curls up on the ground.

Imagine that you fall ill. **Your path to recovery depends on your attitude.** You could complain about the pain or that you feel weak, asking yourself where on earth you could have caught that thing or from whom. Or you could go to a physician, look for useful advice on the Internet, take measures to avoid it happening again. You see the difference. You accept that you are ill. You are not angry, bitter or resentful, but that doesn't mean you are going to do nothing to help yourself get better.

Through acceptance, you get rid of your useless feelings of bitterness and anger which consume your attention and your energy. The time you spend in a temper or feeling sorry for yourself because of your blasted stutter is time wasted. Acceptance is proof of maturity; you can restart from a solid base in a positive frame of mind.

John Steggles, an Australian blogger (Stuttering Jack[3]), has written a superb reply to a young girl who despaired of ever overcoming her stutter.

Firstly, what you must do is accept what is. You will never be able to change until you first deeply and completely accept the situation, and learn to fully love yourself as you are. Take full responsibility for your situation. **You are not a victim to be washed around by the tides of life. It's within your power to change, and the answers for YOU are all out there to be discovered.** You just have to seek them out, and it will be the journey, not the destination, that will nourish your soul.

Love yourself and love everyone you speak to, as this alone, will help wash away the fear of communicating with others.

Acceptance is essential because it replaces the anger, frustration and guilt in your heart with peace, mellowness and serenity. So, who do you think will be the best companions to take with you on the road to communicating freely?

---

[3] stutteringjack.com

I WISH I HAD KNOWN THAT TO ACCEPT

DOESN'T MEAN TO GIVE UP

Yes, I know, perhaps you gritted your teeth when you read the word 'acceptance' in the last chapter.

It's true, **acceptance is often synonymous with resignation** and many people refuse to envisage what they see as an easy way out, an abdication, a pitiful solution to the problem of stuttering.

I am reminded of one message in particular from a mother who explained how her husband couldn't understand their son's attitude. The son had dared to stutter and talk about it at school for the first time. The father was taken aback and said to his son: "That's not like you. You must fight stuttering, not accept it!"

The father had confused acceptance and resignation. **Resignation is a passive attitude. It implies putting up with something that cannot be changed.** A person who resigns himself to his fate would like things to be different but, because he feels powerless, he abandons hope and gives up. So resignation contains two denials: denial of reality and denial of the possibility of action (I've pinched this from somewhere, but I can't remember where). By not acknowledging the problem, you are wasting your time and energy with negative thoughts and behaviors that are totally useless.

Denise Desjardins, author of *Le Bonheur d'Être Soi-même* (*The Joy of Being Yourself*) also explains in an interview that 'acceptance doesn't mean resignation'.

As a child I was already in revolt: against my family's bourgeois life-style, against its religious rites which I thought devoid of meaning, and against my mother, a housewife, who represented everything I wanted to escape from. Much later, when I started to work with Swâmi Prajnânpad, every time I told him of my problems, he replied: 'Accept, accept.' I couldn't stand the word. One day I said to him: 'Acceptance is a sign of weakness, abdication, spineless resignation, defeat. It's a cop-out. And above all it inhibits change. So stop telling me to accept; I can't ever do that.

He then explained that acceptance would allow me to stop fighting with everything and everyone. That my denial would never bring me peace or happiness. **He added that acceptance, when fully understood, could be truly dynamic.**

'Dynamic'. There's an essential adjective for understanding the virtues of Acceptance. By accepting that you are someone who stutters you are not accepting a fixed situation that you are stuck with forever. It is just your present condition. Later, you will be able to progress to the stage where you are working on fluency, and then to the stage where you can speak the way you would like. It is merely a starting block, but finding it is essential if you want to participate in the race.

Bérenger, a fellow blogger (www.jebegaie.com), has also defined acceptance on the Facebook page of his blog:

For me, 'accepting' my stutter is getting to the point where I am completely immune to all the negative aspects of my stuttering. But that doesn't mean doing nothing to get over it. **Accepting your stutter isn't being resigned to it. Accepting means understanding how it works so you can live with it and control it better.**

Lee Reeves, whom I quoted in the last chapter, is on the same wavelength:

> The concept of acceptance does not mean that we are destined to remain at or even be satisfied with the condition in which we find ourselves. It does mean, however, that we have reached a point where we can make clear decisions on our own behalf without the baggage of the past holding us back or the blind optimism of the future jading our expectations for 'perfect' speech. The decision to change the way we speak requires personal risk and will be met with both success and failure. **However, with a foundation of acceptance, success is more sustainable and failure is less destructive.**

In order to illustrate the essential difference between acceptance and resignation, I want to relate a personal anecdote; it concerns you directly because it is related to the writing of this book. Acceptance has greatly helped me to write it. Yes, really! At one time, I was completely snowed under with umpteen notes which I couldn't manage to organize in a coherent way. I could vaguely distinguish where I wanted to go, but I couldn't clearly see how to get there. I almost threw my hands up in despair. I even thought of publishing my notes just as they were, telling readers to work it out for themselves. And then I saw the light.

I accepted that the subject was difficult.

I accepted that the solution wouldn't appear by magic and that the words wouldn't appear on my computer screen automatically and without effort. I accepted that I needed to devise a strategy, an action plan with intermediate objectives so that I didn't become discouraged. I accepted that it would take time.

I accepted that the book wouldn't be perfect.

So, do you think I surrendered in accepting all that? Of course not. It would have been surrendering if I had said to myself that it was too difficult, that I would never manage it; and I wouldn't have persevered.

Instead of that, it really helped to accept the difficulties I would encounter and, as a bonus, I found a simple concrete example of what I wanted to explain. Result: I have succeeded in writing my book and now I am very happy with the finished work with all its imperfections.

I WISH I HAD KNOWN THAT OTHERS WILL REACT TO MY STUTTERING THE WAY I REACT TO IT MYSELF

Changing the way you see and live with your stutter will have a beneficial impact on your state of mind and also on that of people you meet.

This is, in fact, one of the most astonishing discoveries I have made. Other people's reactions were not directly linked to my stuttering but to the way I coped with it and to the image I projected.

If I was embarrassed, they were too. On the other hand, if I looked them in the eye and made reassuring gestures everything went well. People's reactions are merely the reflection of our own emotions. Try smiling at everyone you meet today. You will be surprised.

This is why it is essential to get rid of feelings of shame or guilt. Doing this will allow you to progress and will also have a positive effect on your entourage.

Like Bill Murphy,[4] you will be surprised to see the positive influence of your new way of living with your stutter:

I forced myself to talk to friends about stuttering and learned it was not so much the actual stuttering that bothered them, but rather the evident embarrassment, anxiety and inability to discuss stuttering openly. After much trial and error, I became proficient discussing disfluencies in appropriate social discourse. When I openly shared my stuttering, this put most listeners at ease. They asked questions about stuttering; people were interested, not revolted. When I chose to self-disclose stuttering, the secret was out and I was less tense and fearful. The more stuttering was discussed, the less shame, guilt, and anxiety were experienced. Voluntary exposure quiets these emotions.

Peter Ramig[5] also evokes the pleasure of breaking this taboo, this 'silent conspiracy':

Unsurprisingly, family, friends, and co-workers know we stutter, and are usually unsure of whether or not to maintain eye contact, look away, or fill in the words,

---

[4] American therapist who has stuttered himself. He is one of the authors of *Advice to Those Who Stutter.*
[5] idem

etc. Such uncertainty may create uneasiness and discomfort in our listeners as well as ourselves.

However, much of the uneasiness and uncertainty experienced by both of us can be significantly reduced by acknowledging in an open and matter of fact manner that we stutter. For example, say something as simple as, 'By the way, I'm going to use this opportunity to practice some speech techniques I've been working on lately. This is not an easy chore, but I know you understand why it is important for me to take this opportunity to practice as we speak.' This sample remark gives our listeners an opportunity to ask questions about stuttering, a communication problem that many people find intriguing... Disclosure is a proactive strategy that affords us the opportunity to address our stuttering in a matter of fact and nonchalant manner. **Doing so increases our comfort level because we begin to view our problem in a more positive light.**

Oh yes! Despite what you might think, openly acknowledging your stuttering in front of others is not very difficult. All you have to do is say things simply and just comment on the obvious, as Robert W. Quesal explains very well:

For example, suppose you've met someone for the first time and are making small talk and you're not as fluent as you'd like to be – make a comment about your difficulty: 'Gee, my stuttering seems to be pretty bad today.' Or, 'You'll have to forgive me, I normally don't stutter this much when I meet new people.' This is what my colleague and friend Bill Murphy refers to as 'normalizing' stuttering. Try to accept stuttering as part of you, like your hair color, eye color, height, athletic abilities, writing skills, and any number of other attributes.

Accepting your difference is not only a question of your ability to talk about your stutter, but is also connected to your behavior, as Joseph Sheehan writes:

Next time you go into a store or answer the telephone, see how much you can go ahead in the face of fear. See if you can accept the stuttering blocks you will have more calmly so that your listener can do the same, and in all other situations see if you can begin to accept openly the role of someone who will for a time stutter and have fears and blocks in his speech. But show everyone that you don't intend to let your stuttering keep you from taking part in life. Express yourself in every way possible and practical. **Don't let**

your stuttering get between you and the other
person.

I WISH I HAD KNOWN THAT YOU MUST LOOK YOUR STUTTERING IN THE EYE

Let me tell you about a simple technique which will make your shame vanish and also help you maintain the link with people you talk to. Many 'anti-stuttering' therapies underline **the importance of working on visual contact.** In fact, people who stutter tend to look away when they repeat a sound or block on a word.

Try to maintain eye contact with your listeners. Looking away severs the communication link with your audience and convinces them that you are ashamed and disgusted with the way that you talk.

Gerald R. Moses – Associate Professor of Speech Pathology Eastern Michigan University, Ypsilanti)

Maintaining eye contact will not of itself stop your stuttering, but it will help reduce feelings of shyness and tend to build self-confidence.

Malcolm Fraser

No need to spend five years in analysis to understand (you see, I'm even saving you money): looking away is a way of protecting yourself, to avoid confronting something you don't wish to see. You look away because you perceive stuttering as something 'bad', shameful, and you don't want to see the embarrassment, impatience or pity on the face of the person facing you.

The problem is that by doing this you get exactly the opposite effect. Looking away is taken as a sign of embarrassment and shame. People who find maintaining eye contact difficult, and not only those who stutter, give the impression of being nervous, lacking in self-confidence. As a result, they make the other person ill-at-ease. In looking away, you evoke embarrassment by indicating that something is wrong.

Here are two examples that show how this can destabilize others. The first is a story I found on a forum. In this case the young woman doesn't stutter.

If I am uncomfortable it isn't because I think that stuttering is embarrassing or shameful! It's because the person who is talking to me is embarrassed. My reaction is to look away in the same way as I would look away from something which would make my friend uneasy. It's a classic social reaction: 'it's nothing, in fact I haven't even noticed' (a sneeze, for example, or a tomato sauce stain on a shirt). **On the other hand, I am not embarrassed by my boss' stutter because he openly acknowledges it and continues to maintain eye contact even when he trips over his words.**

The American therapist Tim Mackesey gives another example. He explains that he was being consulted by an 18-year-old with a stutter and his parents. The son explained how he looked away when he addressed his parents because he thought they were embarrassed when he blocked. And the parents explained that they looked away when their son stuttered to avoid putting pressure on him[6]. If that isn't a vicious circle, I don't know what is! And, as if by chance, the son's worst blocks were when he talked to his parents. In just a few days of working on visual contact, the family made considerable progress.

Contrary to what many people who stutter think, communication isn't just a question of words. **It is also a question of gesture, facial expression and**

---

[6] http://www.masteringstuttering.com/there-is-much-more-than-meets-the-eye-contact/

visual contact. The last factor is very important: you use your eyes to capture attention, you use them to convey emotion, and you use them to check that you are being understood, allowing you to adapt to the other person's reactions. Visual contact helps to maintain the conversation, to encourage other people to express themselves, to show that you are listening attentively, to observe body language... and to finish the conversation.

That's the key! If you shut your eyes or look away you cut through the lines of communication. Hardly surprising because, of the four vectors of communication cited above, you have cut three: words, visual contact, and facial expression if you turn your head away at the same time. So you are left with gestures. In that case, unless you happen to be ace at hip-hop or belly dancing, you have to admit that your chances of maintaining contact are somewhat limited.

If you look away, the only thing that remains is your speech block; the other person is left bereft, not knowing how to react. On the other hand, if you smile and maintain visual contact, your stutter will be less noticeable. If you are really stuck, you can reassure with your eyes and show that the interruption is only momentary and that you will take control again. If there is one thing that I have learned about stuttering, it is that everything goes much better if you consider the other person as a partner rather than a judge or an enemy. By maintaining eye contact, you maintain the relationship; you can even initiate a moment of sharing around your speech block.

Visual contact is the thread linking you to the other person. Thanks to this thread, you are showing them that the conversation is continuing and that if they wait just a moment the words will follow. If the visual contact tells them that all is well, that you feel fine, they will feel comfortable too.

Tim Mackesey uses a simple exercise to make his patients understand this. He starts by saying his name: "My name is T-T-T-T-Tim", stuttering but keeping visual contact. Then he says the same words keeping visual contact at first: "My name is..." – at which point he turns his eyes away – "T-T-T-T-Tim". Afterwards, he asks his patients which version left them more at ease. Inevitably they reply: "When you maintained visual contact." And when Tim asks them what they thought when he looked away, they reply: "That you were afraid, uncomfortable." You can try this with a friend: as you will see, it is most edifying.

As Malcolm Fraser said:

> By maintaining eye contact you can demonstrate that you are accepting – not rejecting – your stuttering as a problem to be solved. When you look away, you are denying the problem.

Looking the other person in the eye is also a way of facing up to your stuttering and thus accepting it. But if you turn away you are fleeing yet again, hiding behind a mask, avoiding the problem, perhaps even accepting defeat. Not an ideal way to boost your morale, isn't it?

Maintaining eye contact is therefore a positive step, a way of affirming yourself, a way of holding your head high and reinforcing your confidence. Let's listen to Harold B Starbuck - Distinguished Service Emeritus, Professor Speech Pathology State University College, Geneseo, New York:

> The value of eye contact is the effect it has on the stutterer. It almost forces him to keep the stuttering

going forward through the word. It's an assertive behavior and a positive act. It's hard to withdraw and back off if you are holding eye contact.

In *Self-Therapy for the Stutterer*, Malcolm Fraser, founder of the Stuttering Foundation of America, recommends the following exercises:

Start by looking at yourself in the mirror when alone and faking an easy block. Do you keep eye contact with yourself or do you avert your eyes? Try this repeatedly, making sure that you don't look away. Then do it when making a severe block. If you find you do not keep eye contact before and during the block, work at it until you find that you can and continue doing it.

Then make some phone calls looking at yourself in the mirror while you are having real blocks. Watch yourself until you can talk without shifting your eyes during five or more real stutterings. To complete this program successfully, this is a necessary step.

You can also use visualization. Relax as much as you can and then think of someone you find difficult to look in the eye. Imagine now that you are talking to that person and maintaining visual contact without the least embarrassment and that you even feel pleased about it. This will allow you to prepare yourself confidently.

In a real-life situation, this is how it works:

Establish visual contact before starting to speak.

Two or three seconds of quiet eye contact can get you off to a better start.

Joseph Sheehan

The visual contact must stay natural. Don't stare like a hypnotist; there's no better way to make someone uneasy. You don't need to imitate Kaa (and don't tell me you've never seen 'Jungle Book'). Keeping visual contact does not mean staring someone in the eye but maintaining a balance between looking them in the eye and looking elsewhere.

To stay natural you can look at different areas of their face. This avoids the staring, frenzied look of a psychopath. From time to time you can look to the side but never lower your eyes. This signifies that you have finished the conversation.

If the block lasts too long, you can fall back on a little smile, enough to say "don't panic, I'll get there" to reassure and to play down the situation.

As always, the more you practice the more you will gain confidence, and it will be easier to maintain visual contact as a matter of course when you speak, and above all when you stutter.

In summary, by maintaining visual contact:

- you accept your stutter and live with it better,

- you reinforce your self-confidence by asserting yourself and fighting any feeling of discomfort or inferiority,

- You reinforce your capacity to communicate,

- You make the other person feel at ease and you maintain communication.

It would be a pity to miss out, wouldn't it?

I WISH I HAD KNOWN THAT SPEAKING OPENLY ABOUT MY STUTTERING COULD BE SUCH A RELIEF

The summer 2016 edition of the Stuttering Foundation's magazine contained an article by John Moore, former Director of Marketing for Starbucks. Despite his stutter he has become a consultant and public speaker. He gave advice on talking to an audience. This was his first tip:

Advertise your stutter. Those who stutter know that stuttering happens as a result of trying not to stutter. We focus so much of our mental and physical energy to not stutter that it only heightens our anxiety when speaking. And that results in stuttering. I've found it very helpful to mention my stutter at the start of every presentation I give. Not only does it disarm the audience, it also allows me, the stutterer, the freedom to stutter without shame.

He couldn't be more right. Stop hiding your stutter: bring it out into the open and talk about it! You will be surprised by how receptive people are; by their evident interest, empathy, admiration and encouragement. Don't be afraid to take the first step; there are no hitches and I can see at least three benefits:

1. It changes your ideas about the way your speech is perceived

Are you afraid that your revelation will embarrass people or that they will scoff at you? Believe me, that is exactly the opposite of what happens. At one time, when I was briefly trying out a technique recommended by an ex-stutterer, I talked a little strangely, which intrigued some people. As a result, sometimes I took the initiative and explained what I was doing. I was pleasantly surprised by the reactions which were always positive. This also helped me to stop thinking that stuttering was shameful and something to hide.

2. It is a relief

Why a relief? Because living whilst trying to hide your stutter is both exhausting and frustrating. Indeed, many stutterers make a huge effort to 'hide' their stutter, more or less successfully according to the situation. These 'closet stutterers' are often unnecessarily stressed by their continual need to avoid situations or find subterfuges to escape being unmasked.

Tim Mackesey is a former 'closet stutterer' who has since become a speech therapist. He has a powerful metaphor to describe the consequences of this perpetual disguise:

> For the first thirty years of my life, I **had the impression that I was an undercover cop in the mafia**, living in constant fear of being discovered.

Patricia, whom I met at an International Stuttering Awareness Day held in Marseille told me:

> I was really tired of living under constant pressure, not being able to use the words I wanted, unable to live normally either at home or outside. I felt I had become a prisoner of the system I had created.

So there is only one solution: stop hiding behind a mask. Indeed, people who have decided to lance the abscess and speak openly about their stuttering are unanimous: it is a relief. Patricia whom I just mentioned, for example, went to a group organized by a speech therapist. After three days, she was out on the street, stopping passers-by for a survey asking them what they thought about stuttering! This is how she felt about it:

I had never talked to anybody and all of a sudden I was there explaining to a perfect stranger that I stuttered! When I had completed the first questionnaire, I was so happy that I wanted to shout out loud and jump up and down!

By talking openly about your stutter you will no longer have the impression of running away or hiding. I recall reading this on a forum for stutterers:

For me the turning point was when I admitted before doing a presentation that I had a problem with stuttering. What a relief it was to be able to say those words!

When I first met the woman who was to become my wife, rather than trying to hide and pretend to be 'normal', I took the risk of revealing my stutter straight away. I could be 'natural' and not fear being 'unmasked'. At any rate, it is much more original than "are you still living with your parents?" We are now married, and have three adorable children.

3. It reassures the person you are talking with

In my case, people didn't necessarily understand that I stuttered. They had the impression that I was highly stressed, or that I had a tic. For them, this revelation came as a relief. It's only a stutter!

You need to be aware that, for many people, stuttering is unnerving. They don't know how to behave when faced with someone who stutters. Talking about it gives them the opportunity to ask questions. It also allows you to outline the techniques you have learnt and to be completely free to practice them.

Remind yourself of this: it is not your fault! **You are not admitting to doing something wrong.** The aim isn't to make people sorry for you. Honestly, I don't think I have ever encountered compassion when I have spoken of stuttering; interest, yes, but not compassion.

Their lack of comprehension may even be transformed into a kind of admiration for the fact that you manage – despite everything – to overcome your stuttering and pursue your education or advance in your career.

This transparent approach is a valuable open sesame in situations we fear like oral exams, telephone calls, job interviews, etc.

Thus, it is important to get into the habit early on so the benefits can be recognized. **For example, children may do a presentation at school explaining their stuttering**. This is what Laure did in 6th Grade, aged eleven. Afterwards, she wrote on my blog:

> The morning passed as usual except that I was feeling brave and hopeful. Then finally the moment arrived when I had to give my talk. I was both anxious and excited as I went up to the chalkboard with Julie following close behind. I said to myself: 'Go for it!' and I began. It was as if I was exposing a part of my body but I felt good about it. At the end they applauded us. I was very happy about it. Many other people have done the

same and I hope that people who stutter will follow our example.

From the opposite point of view, that of a teacher, being honest is also to be recommended. Gilles has been teaching for four years. He is 27. He has decided to talk frankly about his speech problem and has stuck to that decision. He believes that if he explains his stutter to his pupils, it will be more difficult for them to use it against him subsequently.

Since I am open and honest on the subject and I don't make a big thing about hiding it, they can't mock me.

He also asks his pupils to help him:

My stuttering mainly involves blocking on certain words. When this happens on a new word that I have to explain, I write it on the chalkboard and just say: 'that's the word. I can't say it so you will have to help me to bring it out'.

I'm overstressing this point because I know that your reaction will be to block; you will be reluctant

to apply my advice. Jim McClure[7] was like you (and like me) but has since changed his mind:

> That desensitizes both you and your listener and, in turn, reduces your tension and helps you speak more fluently. For me, however, putting this compelling logic into practice has been easier said than done. One barrier to advertising has been that like most of us, I grew up believing that stuttering is a bad thing to do. Even though I am getting more proficient at bringing my stuttering out in the open, there's still a voice somewhere in my head shouting 'ARE YOU INSANE? STUTTERING IS BAD! DON'T DO THIS!' I now mention my stuttering without fail whenever I'm in a public speaking situation. This vaccinates both my listeners and me. People often react nervously to stuttering because at first they don't know what's going on. That's especially true for me because my stuttering typically takes the form of silent blocks instead of the repetitions usually associated with stuttering. Mentioning my stuttering up front lets my audience know that if I suddenly freeze in mid-syllable, nothing is amiss: I'm merely stuttering.

Alexandre says the same thing on a forum for people who stutter:

---

[7] http://www.mnsu.edu/comdis/isad6/papers/advertising6.html

In situations where you are certain to stutter, I think that admitting it from the start really saves the day. It lets you relax immediately and set off more confidently. You can say something like: 'I want to tell you that I stutter a little in stressful situations.' The Human Resources Manager will undoubtedly say that there is no reason to be stressed and will be more patient should you stutter. It will also avoid startled looks, with people wondering what is going on when you start to block.

Personally, I've always found it a very difficult thing to say. But sometimes it has helped me immensely, in particular when I had to give a public presentation of an end-of-course project. The fact that I had said that I stuttered left me completely relaxed. As a result I hardly stuttered at all throughout the hour and a half of talking.

When I speak at public meetings on stuttering and explain the necessity of talking openly, there is nearly always a hand in the air – someone wants to confirm the positive reception of this approach. Moreover, nobody has ever contradicted me on this point.

In fact, that's not quite true. It happened once. I was in Nice when a man addressed me. He was a judge with responsibility for applying sentences. Part of his job was to announce the details to the person convicted. And he didn't think that publicizing his stutter would make things easier. No way! So, you see, there are always exceptions. But who knows, perhaps he has since changed his mind.

On the other hand, many people relate how they regret not having dared to speak out. As in the case of Lieven,[8] a medical student:

> At the end of my medical curriculum, there was an oral test attended by a large number of other students. At that moment, I had built up a rather fluent small-talk pattern in the presence of friends, therefore, they were astonished to hear a long silence when simple questions where addressed to me. I blocked totally. The Professor reacted to my distorted face with the suggestion to call the emergency team of the hospital, so augmenting the hilarity of the moment. A short letter to this person or to the ombudsman at the beginning of the year would have been sufficient to avoid this horrible scene!

I agree wholeheartedly with Lieven. It reminds me of an English oral test that I took when I was competing for a place at business school. Although I

---

[8] http://www.mnsu.edu/comdis/isad2/papers/grommen.html

was passably good at the subject, I was almost incapable of bringing out a full sentence in front of the examiner. She took my numerous silences and repetitions as hesitations and a sign of lack of vocabulary. Of course I was marked down badly. As it happens the examiner's husband was my English teacher. When I talked to him about the marks, I said "I don't understand", to which he replied "nor did she".

I should have remembered my French baccalaureate exam which was exactly the opposite experience. My mother had informed the examining board of my stutter and as a result I had been given an extra thirty minutes for the oral test. **What helped me most was that the examiner knew that I stuttered.** This liberated me from my shackles so much that at the end he wanted to know why I had asked for special consideration.

You are also strongly advised to be open about your stutter at job interviews. A few years ago, I applied for a job as marketing manager for a large company. At every interview – with the recruitment agency, then with the Human Resources Manager and finally with my future boss – I said that I stuttered. I knew full well that stuttering could return annoyingly in stressful situations, so I preferred to anticipate. It wasn't a problem. They thanked me for being frank and it relaxed the atmosphere. They could also see from my CV that it had not hindered my professional development, with the result that I was offered the job... although in the end I refused it, but that's another story.

On the other hand, if you manage to get through the interviews by hiding your stutter, the pressure on you will be even stronger when you take up the post or when you start the new course. "Oh God, above all else, they mustn't find out that I stutter, that I've hidden something from them."

Remember too that one percent of the population stutters, which means one applicant in a hundred. You definitely won't be the first stutterer that the examiner or recruiter has met. On the other hand, you will be one of the few who dare speak openly about it, which will certainly be appreciated. Besides, **it might also be an opportunity to showcase the qualities you have needed for your re-education:** willpower, perseverance, rigor, etc. As William, applying for a job as a salesman, said after announcing his stutter: **"it proves I like a challenge"**.

Having established the ground rules, here are some simple recommendations for putting them into practice.

1. **You don't need to get into a long and detailed explanation.** You are not a stutterer above all else, and also other people attach much less importance to it than you do. Be satisfied with the facts and present them without fuss.

2. **You don't need to make excuses.** Stuttering isn't a fault and even less your fault. It exists, that's all.

> Don't apologize for your speech. Your stuttering is a part of you. Saying, 'sorry but I stutter' is like me getting up and saying, 'sorry guys, but I am a woman. How wrong would that be?
>
> Nina G.

3. **You are not announcing the death of your grandmother, only saying that you stutter.** Keep smiling and relax. Don't hesitate to joke about it. It is

your business to set the tone. If you seem embarrassed everyone else will too. If you speak in a relaxed way, the listener will take in the information, may possibly be inclined to ask a couple of questions, and will then pass quickly onto another subject.

I can well understand that you may feel reticent about initiating the conversation by announcing out of the blue that you stutter. So here is Tom's story, taken from the Neurosemantics[9] forum. Tom makes it a point of honor that stuttering is not the first thing he talks about. This is how he does it:

Hello, I'm Tom. [Then I say something about myself which has nothing to do with stuttering, so it isn't the first thing I highlight.] By the way, I stutter which is why I speak like that...

He insists on saying "I speak like that" rather than "I speak badly or I have difficulty in speaking" or other possibilities, because they imply a judgement on stuttering. He restricts himself to recognizing the existence of his stutter and announces it as a fact.

---

[9] Forum for stutterers who find cognitive and behavioral therapies useful.

Nevertheless, if this approach still seems too direct to you, you can wait for the first block. Alexandre explains:

Without saying that you stutter, you can simply say something reassuring the first time you block, such as: 'Oh! Those words just won't come out this morning'. Something anyone might say when they get tongue-tied. It lets you calm down and releases the pressure so that you can progress.

John, who is also a contributor to the Neurosemantics forum, agrees:

The first time you block you can say something like: 'By the way, I would just like to say that I stutter sometimes and that I am working on it. So I may struggle with some words, like just now', said perfectly naturally whilst keeping good eye contact. Remember the rule: people will take their lead from the way you act yourself. So by acting like this you are programming their reaction.

You can also do it on the telephone. Yet again, being frank is a way of avoiding awkwardness and incomprehension. Let's listen in on Joe. He had to call the after-sales service because his computer was broken:

I knew it was going to be a long conversation so I was upfront about things, telling the man on the help-desk: 'Hello, I want to ask some questions but firstly I would like to warn you that I stutter. So don't worry if there are some unusually long silences when I speak [I normally have silent blocks]'. The guy was cool about it and replied in a sympathetic tone: 'OK'. **Announcing my stutter greatly reduces the tension in the conversation so I try to use this strategy as often as possible.** Despite that, I don't want to give the impression that I am apologizing, so I never say 'Sorry, but I stutter.'

I would like to conclude on this essential step in your journey with a tale Ryme related on my blog:

Hi, I have an exclusive scoop for you. I am pleased to announce that my oral went very well. I said right at the beginning that I had a problem with stuttering and so I was under much less pressure. Yes, I stuttered on a few words, but not much, and that's all. I even had the strength and the courage to put down my notes and improvise everything... Above all, I said what I wanted to say, when I wanted to, and that is priceless...

I can confirm that: the ability to be oneself and to show your real self is invaluable.

I WISH I HAD KNOWN THAT STUTTERING RESPONDS POSITIVELY TO HUMOR!

According to Fred Murray, one of the contributors to *Advice to Those Who Stutter* and author of *A Stutterer's Story,* these are the three most important pieces of advice he has been given:

Stop worrying about yourself and your stuttering. You are too focused on it.

Find a project you can throw yourself into, something creative which will help other people.

And above all, keep your sense of humor.

Fred is absolutely right. **When it's time to let the cat out of the bag and reveal your stuttering, humor and self-derision are particularly effective weapons.**

When it comes to poking fun at herself, Nina G is a true professional, presenting herself as she does as 'the only comedian who stutters'. As an American stand-up comedian, she has confounded those who said she could never take to the stage. For some time now she has even been teaching courses on public speaking. This is what she has to say about talking about her stuttering:[10]

> I personally, disclose my stuttering in stand-up comedy or when doing presentations as early as possible: 'just so you know, I stutter so you are going to have to wait for all of the brilliant things I have to say.' This usually breaks the ice plus I just told the people I am meeting with how I want them to respond to my speech and that I am a capable person. The reality is that most people don't know how to respond to our speech since we might be the first person they have ever met who stutters. If we can mold their response to us it can save some awkward moments later on.

> Everyone is going to disclose their stuttering differently. You should develop a way that you are comfortable with and even try it out on different friends and family to see their response. Remember, it is your stuttering, your presentation and your audience. So many times as people who stutter we feel our speech is

---

[10] https://ninagcomedian.wordpress.com/2015/01/18/five-tips-for-stuttering-your-way-through-presentations/

out of our control. When doing presentations, you may not have control of your stuttering, but you do have control over your presentation so seize it!

David tells the story of when he took a course for Christians converting to Catholicism:

> I blocked on 'Methodist' for probably a full minute, finally stopped, and stated that 'I am converting because I find Catholic much easier to say!', then proceeded with the original word. The effect was wonderful. I had acknowledged to everyone at the table that there was in fact something out of the norm going on, that I was aware of it, and most importantly that it was OK to talk about, which we subsequently did.[11]

When you adopt this attitude you will make people laugh: they aren't laughing *at* you but *with* you. And that makes all the difference. As Charles Van Riper said: "Humor and negative emotion can't sleep in the same bed".

You won't necessarily be able to joke about stuttering straight away, but when you do it will be a very good sign.

---

[11] You can read many others examples of 'stuttering humor' on the Stuttering Home Page http://www.mnsu.edu/comdis/kuster/humor.html

One mother, writing on an Internet forum, had this to say on the subject:

This morning, as he was getting up, my four-and-a-half-year-old son said to me [elongating words is his way of speaking]:

'Mmmmmummmy, I speak like a cow' [going moo].

I didn't dare say anything but he burst out laughing. Later, he asked me why I didn't laugh. I said that I didn't want to make fun of him. He replied:

'It isn't making fun of me but making fun of my stutter.'

And he continued to laugh.

You see? At four and a half, this child already had the best possible reaction to his stutter: he accepted it, made jokes about it, and didn't feel guilty or ashamed; and he knew that stuttering was only one part of him. He'll go a long way that kid!

Humor also works very well as a chat-up line. In this discipline Mark must be the champion in all categories: he has completely reversed the situation by transforming his stutter from a stumbling block into an original way of approaching someone he finds attractive. He even manages to present it so that if he stutters it will not only be understood but also appreciated! It would be difficult to find a better way of releasing the pressure. Here's how he goes about it:

Hello. I'm Mark and I would really like to get to know you. There's only one thing: I stutter... and the prettier the girl is, the more I stutter!

World champion!

I WISH I HAD KNOWN THAT EVERY AVOIDANCE IS A WASTE OF TIME AND THAT YOU MUST NEVER LET STUTTERING PREVENT YOU FROM MOVING FORWARD

Avoidance is the preferred hobby of people who stutter. **It can take several forms:** substituting one word for another, inserting unwanted fillers (um, err...), verbal tics, or throat clearing. It could be a telephone you don't answer (or pretend not to hear), a question you don't ask or a reply you don't give. Sometimes it might be a funny story that you don't tell because you are too afraid of getting stuck on the punchline. It could be a touch of humor that you might have added to a conversation or a proposition that you keep to yourself...

My earliest memory of avoidance goes back to my childhood. My mother had asked me to buy some Ajax at the corner shop. The first thing I thought of was the letter A of Ajax, like a red light being switched on in my brain. That letter A was an obstacle that had been placed in my path. On the road to the shop, that A continued to grow, becoming so terribly big so that when I stood in front of the shopkeeper I asked for Persil. Just to avoid taking on that terrible A.

All those words held back or avoided engender a passing relief but finish by burning a hole in your guts just as surely as acid would. In the long term you become disheartened. **Little by little these avoidances become second nature. The effects can go a very long way, dictating even the most insignificant decisions.** The apprehension may thus transform itself into fear and then a real phobia.

Some people go so far as to pretend they are dumb or have lost their voice in certain situations, or assert that they are ill when faced with an oral exam or a presentation. Another example: in a restaurant you choose a dish that you will be able to pronounce rather than the one you would really like. That may seem laughable, but when it ends up having an impact on your life choices, it is much more serious. You may avoid studying certain subjects (sales, media studies, etc.) or refuse to apply for a job where you have to talk in public or answer the telephone, then refuse a church wedding to avoid saying your vows in public and so on. As Joseph Sheehan wrote: **"avoidance is a toboggan ride to failure"**.

Therefore, the first commandment of someone who stutters should be: "Thou shalt not fall into the temptation to substitute a word; nor shalt thou avoid opportunities for speaking".

It is this avoidance that maintains your shame, your fear and your low self-esteem. I have read somewhere that in order to feel proud of yourself it is sufficient to do things of which you are proud. I would add: and stop doing things of which you are not proud. Evidently avoiding words and remaining silent when you have something to say fall into that category.

You mustn't let stuttering dictate your behavior and your life in general any longer. This resolution is undoubtedly of prime importance. As Alexandre wrote on an Internet forum:

When you are thinking of doing something, ask yourself a question: am I hesitating because of my stutter? If the answer is yes, then do it. **Otherwise you are letting stuttering dictate what you can and cannot do; you are letting it take over.**

Joe is American and president of a local association for people who stutter. When he was a child, Joe had a serious stutter. He blocked frequently, he suffered from tics and, of course, he avoided situations where he would have to talk. But there came a time when he decided that instead of whining and cursing his fate he would consider his stutter to be a friend: "I turned around," Joe explains, "and said, come here buddy!"

That was the moment he swore that he would stop making decisions based on his stuttering. Since then, rather than waiting to be able to say things 'properly' before doing something, he just does it. Nowadays he has a very slight stutter but he talks so much and is so expressive into the bargain that it isn't noticeable. The only thing he did was to eradicate avoidance, pressure and fear. Joe isn't an eminent theorist on the subject of stuttering but he has something important to say: **"We start with a small stutter, but it is we who make it so big."**

Alan Badmington, a retired policeman from Wales, had a pronounced stutter and had become a past master in the art of avoidance.

I had particular problems with words commencing with the initial letter 'b' (which was unfortunate because my surname is Badmington) but also had difficulty with 'c, d, f, g, j, k, m, n, p, s, t,' and 'v,' to name but a few! Consequently, I avoided such words and substituted them with synonyms not commencing with the dreaded letters!

He tells how, when he stopped an offender in the street, he had to phone in to police control and say where he was. If the name of the street began with a sound that he couldn't pronounce he would drag the offender to another street before calling. At his wedding, he opted to say his vows at the same time as the minister to be sure he wouldn't block. It was a successful strategy but now he jokes that:

There are still a few things that concern me regarding that episode. I frequently lie awake at night, wrestling with the following questions:

Am I married to my wife?

Am I married to the vicar?

Is my wife married to the vicar? or
Are we all three joined in holy matrimony?

Challenging avoidance is a central message in Alan's writing:

Each time we avoid something, we strengthen its influence over us. We can evade for so long, but the time will come when the situation demands that we have to say a specific word, or speak in a particular situation. When that happened, I found that my fear level had increased so much that I stuttered more severely.

So, Alan made a resolution that changed his life: he adopted a policy of zero-tolerance towards all kinds of avoidance: "I vowed that I would never again substitute a word, nor shirk the challenge of any speaking situation."

If a word wouldn't come out, he didn't replace it by another one but instead put into practice what he had learnt about overcoming a block. This strategy was crucial to him daring to face up to his fears - fear of being in a situation where he needed to communicate, fear of saying that he stuttered, fear of using speech therapy techniques, etc. **He chose to see new situations as learning experiences rather than difficulties to be overcome. From that moment his self-image started to improve and he entered into the virtuous circle of increasing confidence.** Today, he is a remarkable speaker, sought out world-wide for lectures on his life story.

Actually, you will feel a sense of achievement by voluntarily seeking out feared words and entering difficult situations. The less you avoid, the more confidence you will have in yourself as a respectable and worthy person.

Malcolm Fraser.

The advantages of this change of attitude can be resumed in this formula: **"If you flee from your fear, it will follow you. Face up to it and it will disappear."**

Indeed, facing up to a situation reinforces your confidence and **creates a virtuous circle** which can be resumed as follows:

"I move forward – I realize that it isn't as difficult as I thought and, even if it is, it is becoming less so – I replace my frustration by the satisfaction of having dared – I have a better self-image – I regain confidence – this confidence allows me to dare try other things – and so on"

This virtuous circle can be found in the stories of numerous people who stutter.

The virtuous circle of speech fluency

Stuttering isn't a fault; I have to be daring in order to progress; I am capable of expressing myself

Release of pressure

Reinforcement of confidence and self esteem

End of avoidance strategies; progressive desensitisation

Satisfaction of having dared; positive experiences

www.goodbye-begaiement.fr

Catherine is a young Polish woman. She has a lovely metaphor for the benefits of this change in attitude:

Say to yourself that you have two houseplants: one is carnivorous, the 'Word Monster', and the other is a 'Yes We Can' plant. **Every time you slip into avoidance you are watering the Word Monster which becomes a little more terrifying** whilst the plant which embodies your self-confidence shrinks. **On the other hand, every time you are courageous you water the Yes We Can plant and you regain confidence.** The aim is to dry up the Word Monster and feed the Yes We Can.

Hal B has been stuttering since primary school. His schooldays were blighted by the mockery of the other children as well as some of his teachers. Nevertheless, one day he found the strength to surmount his fear. He was 15 at the time.[12]

I was slated to give a presentation on a section of Jewish literature for what was supposed to be a small crowd of maybe two dozen people at most. At the end of this presentation, I had to read a rather large section of scripture written in ancient Aramaic, which I wasn't good at reading fluently to say the least. But what was supposed to be a small group turned out to be the entire school. Granted, I went to a small school, so it was only about a hundred people, but I didn't know about this

---

[12] https://themighty.com/2016/03/why-i-chose-to-continue-a-high-school-presentation-when-my-stutter-was-at-its-worst/

change until literally minutes before. All the mental preparation I did for this presentation went out the window. To make a long story short, I stuttered so much that the headmaster actually came up and offered to take over reading the Aramaic for me.

In that moment, I had a choice. I could take the easy way out, or I could fight and finish what I started. I chose to fight, no matter how painful it was, and I finished that presentation, stuttering and all.

They say that sometimes you have to hit rock bottom to find the strength to overcome, and that painful Friday was my rock bottom. I had seen the worst my stutter could throw at me that day. The public humiliation of my ordeal was so great that part of my mind begged me to never speak in public again. And if I never spoke in public after that, who could really blame me?

But I refused to allow my stutter to limit me, remembering the hundred pairs of pitying eyes in the audience on that awful day and vowing to never let that happen again. I fought. I fought through every stutter and every block that occurred. And it's a battle that still goes on today. Every day is a new fight, a new battle to win. I'm not successful every day, but each new day is another chance for fluency, and it's a challenge I always greet.

For those who are currently engaged in their own battles, don't give up. Don't let the ones who wish to see you falter through their words and actions dictate how you live your life. For every person who wants to see you fail, there are many more who are rooting for you. Know that the righteous are out there and don't forget their presence even on your darkest days.

In a way I feel blessed. Blessed that I was given a challenge that has taught me the meaning of courage. Blessed that I learned not only patience with myself but patience with others. Blessed that I learned to accept the challenges others face as they accept mine. Blessed that this challenge is teaching me how to overcome fear in order to live a full life.

As the great journalist Dorothy Thompson once said, **"Only when we are no longer afraid do we begin to live.**

It was a decisive moment for Hal. He is now at university studying diplomacy and international affairs. His Yes We Can plant is flourishing.

I WISH I HAD KNOWN THAT YOU DON'T HAVE TO BE GOOD TO START BUT YOU HAVE TO START TO BE GOOD

Despite what I have just said, perhaps you are still hesitating. You think it is too soon, that you are not ready, and so on.

For many years I used to tell myself: "When I stop stuttering, I will do that thing".

It was a big mistake because, without realizing it, I was tackling the problem the wrong way round.

It was only when I decided to adopt the opposite attitude that I started to progress. Actually, you need to 'do that thing' in order to finally stop stuttering. It is through the experience of speaking that you acquire skills and progress. Don't say: "When I no longer stutter, I will use the telephone" but "I will use the telephone so I stop stuttering when I make a call".

Let's pursue this idea. Although most people, whether they stutter or not, panic at the idea of speaking in public, John Moore has created a therapy based on it! He calls himself 'The Stuttering Presenter'.

> For too many years, stuttering stifled my voice and stunted my growth. It wasn't until I reached a very low point in my life that I decided stuttering wasn't going to manage me. Instead, I was going to manage my stuttering. Meaning, I wasn't going to allow the shame and guilt of stuttering to silence my voice. I was going to use every tool I had learned to minimize my disfluency and actively seek opportunities to speak, even if I stuttered. It was simple. For me to stop stuttering, I had to start talking.[13]

He has since come a long way. This is the same John Moore who became Starbucks' Marketing Director. The author of *The Passion Conversation*, he has become a consultant and has more than 250 presentations around the world to his credit.

You know the expression 'diving in at the deep end'? Well, the following example is a good

---

[13] http://www.stutteringhelp.org/content/stuttering-public-speaking

illustration of the principle. Imagine that you are overweight and that, as well as your diet, your physician advises you to go swimming regularly in the local pool. If you are ashamed of your body you won't dare to be seen in a swimming costume and you won't go swimming. By refusing to accept your shape, by refusing to expose your singularity to the light of day, you are denying yourself the possibility of exercise and resolving a part of the problem. It is exactly the same for stuttering. **By refusing to expose yourself to others, you are not putting yourself in situations where you have to talk, situations that will help you put into practice your techniques and increase your self-confidence.**

The most common method used for moving ahead and gaining confidence is called **'progressive desensitization'**. The principle is simple. You list things you are afraid of (words, situations, people, etc.) in order of how apprehensive they make you. **Then you deliberately confront these words or situations, gradually working up from the least frightening ones. The idea is to progressively**

acquire the confidence which will help you when you come to face the next situation.

I like to use a skiing metaphor to illustrate why you need to begin and how this gradual learning scheme works. People who stutter are like those novice skiers who cross their skis and fall every few feet each time they set off down a slope. For them, skiing is exhausting, distressing, dangerous and an excellent way of being made to feel foolish. They see others enjoying themselves, reveling in the sensations and giving the impression that it is easy. Novice skiers can become disheartened and irritated.

Let's imagine that this year you have decided to try skiing. You will book an instructor for private lessons or maybe join a class; or perhaps you will teach yourself by reading manuals written by experts, watching videos of champions and participating in ski forums. But whatever your choice **you won't make any progress until you put on your skis and descend your first slope.**

The first technique you will learn is the snowplow. It is neither very stylish nor very fast but at least it lets you get going without too much risk. You will start with easy slopes, accompanied by your instructor, and improve your skills. Then you will move progressively to more difficult slopes. **You will fall head over heels, sometimes spectacularly. But if you persevere, if you go skiing every day, you will progress, hone your technique, try more difficult slopes** and even go it alone without your instructor. You will be able to bring your skis closer and closer together and do parallel turns. You will become progressively less apprehensive. You will relax, feel at ease and your gestures will become more fluid. You will start to enjoy skiing, feeling that marvelous sensation of gliding down the slopes. Finally you will be skiing without thinking, reveling in the sensations, amazed by the surroundings.

Now reread the above passage replacing 'skis' with 'words', 'skiing' with 'talking' and 'slope' by 'speaking situation'. Amazing isn't it?

As far as I am concerned I'm hardly Olympic standard and I could be more stylish but I'm good enough to enjoy myself and go wherever I want.

And that's the most important thing, isn't it?

I WISH I HAD KNOWN THAT THE SMALLEST ACTION IS BETTER THAN THE NOBLEST INTENTION

Perhaps you have already been looking for some time for information on stuttering.

You have read personal stories and articles on blogs which have inspired you.

You have bought books on stuttering.

You have joined forums and Facebook groups.

And then...

You have reread the articles.

You have read more discussions on social media and in forums.

But you have still haven't done anything!

And you are beginning to feel slightly guilty – the first sign of an upcoming depression – the stage also known as 'I'll do it when I get a round tuit' or, depending on the day, 'Mondayitis'.

I sympathize. I really do. Because I was like you. I am a world champion dabbler. I have an outstanding collection of broken resolutions. And I think that for a long while my failure to 'go for it' slowed any significant progress.

Yes, I admit that sometimes I have the backbone of a jellyfish, and I really admire people who are capable of getting up at five o'clock to do an hour of sport before going to work. I know that this is the main obstacle I face in order to progress and I am sure that it is the same for many other people.

Since you have read a wealth of good advice and the most inspiring of personal stories, you know what you need to do to stop stuttering. **But the real transformation can only happen if you take action.** As the Stuttering Foundation of America points out: "There are many proven, effective ways to reduce stuttering: **doing nothing is not one of them!**"

Let's summarize:

Reading blogs and books isn't taking action

Deciding isn't taking action

Taking action is taking action

The worst thing is that we have known this for a long time. As early as the 8th century, Padmasambhava (known in Tibet as the 'second Buddha' – that's just to let you know that he wasn't just anyone) said: "If you want to know your past life, look at your present condition; if you want to know your future life, look at your present actions." To summarize: **"What you are tomorrow is the result of what you do today."** The only question to ask yourself now is thus: **"Are you doing anything about it?"** And if that isn't the case, how can you get yourself going? How can you change from the verb 'to read' to the verb 'to do'?

You will really start to change your life from the moment you make a decision. And a real decision can be recognized by the fact that you have tried doing something new. If you haven't done anything new, you haven't really made a decision.

According to Anthony Robins, a charismatic personal development guru from the United States:

Knowledge is not power... It's potential power. Execution will trump knowledge any day.

And he's right. Because the worst thing is that, most of the time, you know what you should do. You are fully aware of it.

You know that you should go out, smile and meet other people rather than stay shut up in your bedroom.

You know that you should practice daily the speech fluency techniques you have learnt.

You know that you must practice using the telephone again and again, and stop being afraid of it.

But nevertheless you don't do it. And nothing changes.

Let's go back to the metaphor of learning to ski. If you read books written by experts, watch videos of champions, participate in skiing forums, do you think that, having done all that, you will be able to ski?

I'm not writing this to rub your nose in the dirt. I would like to be reassuring; many people find it difficult to take action. It is one of the commonest subjects on blogs and books dedicated to personal development, which are filled with advice on fighting against our natural tendency to put things off. As the saying goes, 'procrastination is the thief of time'.

My first piece of advice is to **select one resolution only**. This will prevent you from taking on too much. It is much easier, and managing to keep a single resolution is often enough to create a virtuous circle.

Alan Badmington did this. One fine day, he resolved that he would never again dodge a word or an opportunity to speak. He decided to apply a policy of **zero tolerance to avoidance**. This simple but essential rule allowed him to set off on his journey, to dare to face up to his fears, to practice, and to gain in competence and confidence.

Others have chosen to stutter voluntarily, affronting their fear of blocks and repetitions, minimizing their importance and thus taking away a large part of the load which was weighing down their speaking.

The first thing that I myself put into practice successfully was maintaining visual contact. By doing this I was looking my stuttering in the eye, or rather ceasing to look away when I encountered it. This simple change had an influence on my thought patterns, my attitude and my way of communicating. It resulted in a change in perception when I stuttered, both for me and for the person listening.

A well-chosen resolution will allow you to undo the complex knot of your stuttering. Pulling on a loose end will enable you to extract a long length of string from the ball, exposing the next knot, for which you may need to formulate another resolution.

Indeed, if you manage to keep your first resolution, you may eventually add more. **You will benefit from the boost in confidence due to your success with the first resolution.**

Be careful, though, not to confuse goal and good resolution. It's a classic mistake, you brainless nitwits. Let's take an example. You want to lose weight: this is a goal. In order to do so, you will go running twice a week: this is a resolution. With a resolution, we are taking action. If your goal is to no longer faint every time a telephone rings in the vicinity, you will resolve to make at least three calls daily.

The advantage of resolutions is that you have a daily opportunity to keep them. And failing isn't a disaster. As Gretchen Rubin says in her book *The Happiness Project*:

> Every day I try to apply my good resolutions. Sometimes I succeed, sometimes I fail, but each morning I start from scratch.

Are you happy with that? Perhaps there is a question lurking at the back of your mind: "How do I choose my resolution?"

Good question! **Simply choose the one which will have the greatest impact on your stuttering**, the one you are most motivated by. Don't necessarily choose the one which seems the easiest.

Luckily, you have a source of inspiration for good resolutions: other people have already tried and succeeded in their journey to fluency. The list below will help. It comes from strategies mentioned on my blog, used by people who have liberated themselves from their stuttering.

I will talk when I feel like it, stuttering or not.

I will do a presentation on my stutter in class.

I will make all my phone calls myself.

I will no longer replace one word by another; nor will I avoid opportunities to speak.

I will use the fluency techniques that I have learnt (breathing, articulation, managing blocks).

And so on.

An excellent way of keeping a resolution is to announce it to your friends and family. Those who are in the know will encourage you and re-motivate you. Tell your brother or your sister, your best friend, your speech therapist, your nearest and dearest, and so on. You can add extra motivation by promising to do something if you break your resolution: do their housework for a month, make a donation to a political party that you detest, etc. Undoubtedly this will strengthen your determination!

Nowadays, when something displeases me or causes difficulties I automatically ask myself a question. "Am I doing something about it?" Which means, once I have understood the parameters and identified the problem, what am I doing to make things change? Looking for a speech therapist, that's doing something. Talking about stuttering to someone close, that's doing something. Refusing to avoid a word, that's doing something. Picking up the phone to make calls, that's doing something.

I don't know whether it was Gandhi or Donald Duck who said: "If you want to change something in your life you are going to have to do something you have never done" but I quite agree.

And I promise you: in one year's time you will be pleased to have started today.

I WISH I HAD KNOWN THAT BEING POSITIVE AND CHANGING MY THOUGHTS COULD REALLY CHANGE MY LIFE

Changing my state of mind has been a determining factor in my progress. As Voltaire said: "I have chosen to be happy; it's better for my health".

I have learned to abandon my negative thoughts (I will never manage it, I am useless, etc.), which only served to push me deeper into the hole. I chose to think about solutions rather than feel sorry for myself. Instead of saying: "I have to do a presentation. That's terrible: how can I avoid it?" today I say to myself: "How can I best prepare it? How can I handle it?"

As part of his reply to a young girl who stutters, the blogger Stuttering Jack underlines the importance of this transformation.

You must stop using negative affirmations and visualizations. These are powerful forces that are currently working against you rather than in your favor. Instead of negative affirmations like 'life isn't going to get better, it's going to get worse', 'I know there is no cure', 'an improvement will be a miracle', 'a life that will mean nothing to the world' and visualizations like 'I can never see that happening', 'I can't even see getting married', I want you to **use positive affirmations and visualizations that create, in your mind, the pictures and images that you want to see, in your life, even if they seem such a distant dream to you, and keep them in the forefront of your mind, in big and bright colors. See yourself in that ideal picture and feel what it would be like to live that dream.** Do this every day and you will begin to move towards that, even if it seems so far away.

Here are six tips to help you leave the dark side of these forces behind:

Tip no. 1: Be aware of how toxic your thoughts are

Saying that thinking hurts couldn't be truer. Research published by the University of Michigan[14] in 2011, supported by MRI scans, shows that the same areas of the brain are used when you scald yourself on a cup of coffee and when you recall an unhappy love affair. In other words, the brain doesn't distinguish between physical and emotional pain. Your negative thoughts really are toxic and need to be eliminated.

To help you remember this, here is a simple trick taken from Paulo Coelho's book, *Maktub* (yep, I had a Coelho phase too). He explains that you need to displace the pain onto the physical plane in order to understand how bad it is for you.

Dig the nail of your index finger into your thumb every time you have a painful thought. If you transform your negative thoughts into physical pain it will help you understand how bad they are for you. And once you have done that you will be able to avoid them.

So, every time you think "I'm useless. I can't even say what I want to," pinch yourself hard. You should soon get over it.

---

[14] ww.cnn.com/2011/HEALTH/03/28/burn.heartbreak.same.to.brain/index.html

Here is another idea from our friend Paulo to help us recognize our harmful thoughts: give them a human face.

All you have to do is to put all your anxiety, your fear, your disappointments in an invisible being who follows you around everywhere. He plays the part of 'Mr. Nasty' in your life, always proposing attitudes and feelings that are bad for you. Once you have created this avatar, it is easy to avoid following his advice.

My own personal villain looks like Jack Nicholson in 'The Shining'. I can tell you: it works.

Tip no. 2: Socrates' triple filter test

I have bad memories of old man Plato. For a whole summer I had to plow through three or four books on philosophy, including *The Republic*, before the start of term. The holiday pictures are not on my mantelpiece. Plato almost succeeded in putting me off reading for life, and I've had a grudge against him ever since. I never thought I would quote him one day. However, thanks to Plato I have recently discovered that Socrates was already practicing cognitive therapy more than 2000 years ago.

It was Socrates who first said that we should test the validity of our beliefs by means of three filters. So, each time a negative thought tries to spoil your life, you must ask yourself three simple questions:

"Is what I believe absolutely true?" If the answer is no, ask yourself the second question: "Is it useful to believe it?" If the reply is still no, the last question should let you deal a final blow to your negativity (unless you are a real masochist): "Do I like believing it?" Try this exercise with the following: "They will think I am useless" or "I'm going to mess up and be ridiculous". This process should throw considerable doubt onto your convictions so you can pass onto something more constructive.

Tip no. 3: Write down your doubts and fears

Now you have realized that these thoughts are toxic and that they rarely pass through the triple filter test. But how do you get rid of those which keep buzzing around in your head? According to a recent study by Sian Beilock (Chicago University), writing down your worries just before a stressful event (like an exam or a presentation) will boost your performance. Those students who wrote down their fears ten minutes before an exam had significantly better results than those who didn't.

How does she explain this? Worry 'clogs up' the brain and stops it from working at its best. Writing down one's worries unblocks the channels, allowing it to dedicate itself as much as possible to the task in hand. According to the Chicago University researchers, this kind of exercise helps people do their best in 'high pressure' situations like a job interview, an important meeting or speaking in public.

In general, keeping a journal is a good habit. You can note your doubts, your fears and your beliefs, and understand better what there is lurking behind them; and also you can keep a note of your successes. Mark Irwin (President of the International Stuttering Association 2001-2007) advises:[15]

> Record Success. Keep a Journal. Write down when you spoke well (describe who, when and where.) I found reviewing the ever expanding list of successful speaking situations to be extremely powerful in changing my speaking self-image. I think too often people who stutter have over emphasized their limitations as

---

[15] https://www.mnsu.edu/comdis/isad5/papers/irwin.html

communicators. To my mind it is important that this false image be corrected by receiving validation as a speaker wherever possible. The journal helped me do this.

Clément also took to heart the advice to write down his worries before doing a presentation, as he explained on my blog:

A few hours from now, I have to give a presentation before an audience of twenty people. Being a stutterer, naturally I am apprehensive.

I am afraid of blocking frequently, feeling I am being sneered at; I dread being misunderstood, being judged by the public. And also that the public and the teacher will be embarrassed.

But I have things to say. I must and I will say them. I am a human being, not just a stutterer. I am going to concentrate on what I have to say, concentrate on the public and accept that, inevitably, I will block. But the most important thing is that I say what I have to say. And I am going to keep in mind the pleasure one gets from having conveyed the message.

Reading those lines, you can better understand how writing can help. By naming his fears, Clément has also found a way of combatting them, without necessarily thinking he was doing so. And, within the space of a few words, he has leapt from anticipating disaster to a positive image, which helped him to confront the situation more calmly. In fact, he later explained that rereading his note just before his ordeal had greatly helped him.

Tip no. 4: 'Walk the talk' and change your viewpoint

Astonishingly, the best way to acquire a skill is to behave as if you already have it. A recent scientific study has demonstrated the efficacy of 'walking the talk' on self-confidence. According to this study (published in *Psychological Science*, 2010) acting self-confident produces psychological and behavioral changes as well as variations in neuroendocrine levels.

The researchers made one group of subjects adopt open, expansive, high-power postures whilst the second group was asked to mimic the opposite. They discovered that the high-power displays engender an increase in testosterone (associated with assertiveness and risk-taking) and a decrease in cortisol (associated with anxiety and fear). Exactly the inverse was found in those who adopted postures of weakness. Subjects in the first group also said that they felt more powerful and more inclined to take risks.[16]

René, a specialist in NLP and a contributor to a neurosemantics forum,[17] has been able to see the effects of this approach on his patients. He believes that, in order to change your thoughts, you must change your viewpoint, your way of perceiving what is going on. He advises people who are worried about introducing themselves in public, for example at a meeting, to change their viewpoint. Change "I don't want to introduce myself" into "I can't wait to introduce myself".

You need to rediscover your inner child, jumping up and down with impatience because you have to wait for your turn on a fairground carousel. So, before making a telephone call, for example, you could visualize what you would think and feel if you really wanted to do it. As if you had just been given a

---

[16] For more on this subject, I strongly suggest that you watch the Internet video produced by Amy Cuddy, one of the psychologists who participated in the study: 'Your body language shapes who you are".
[17] English-language forum on the application of cognitive and behavioural techniques to stuttering therapy.
https://groups.yahoo.com/neo/groups/neurosemanticsofstuttering/info

present and you were really impatient to tear open the wrapping and discover what was inside.

René writes:

> Your brain cannot tell the difference between what is real and what isn't. So if you pretend to be an excited, happy child, your brain will simply adapt to this view point and generate positive thoughts. Try it, not just once, but at least nine or ten times. You are breaking a habit and that takes time. It's all about knowing how to modify your view point and understanding that, however you may feel, it is the result of what you are thinking at the time.

René not only uses this technique for speaking in public but also for motivating himself to do the housework or take out the rubbish. There's a way of making your partner or your parents happy!

Tip no. 5: pay attention to others

This is a tip given by Tim Mackesey, a former stutterer who has become a speech therapist. He thinks that our nervousness comes from the fact that we are too introverted, too egocentric: Will they like ME? Are they going to mock ME? Will I forget MY words? Will they think I am good? He recommends that rather than thinking about yourself you should focus on your listeners.

I have read a report of how this technique was used successfully by a NLP specialist on a young woman who stuttered. He had noticed that his patient's stuttering was particularly evident when she was in stressful situations. As a way of destressing her, he taught her to focus on what the other people present were doing. His starting point was the basic observation that in order to feel anxious we have to be thinking of ourselves. However, we can't pay attention to our own thoughts, our environment and other people all at the same time. Brenda followed this advice and noticed that she no longer reached the level of anxiety which normally aggravated her stuttering. Another beneficial effect was that it made her more observant of others and because of this she found them less frightening.

This experience reminds me of what Lewis Carroll, author of *Alice in Wonderland* and a very good stutterer to boot, used to say: "If you can't not think about something, it is always possible to think about something else."

Tip no. 6: Be your best own best friend

This is my favorite tip so I've kept it till last.

We tend to focus on setbacks and judgements from outside ourselves whether they are real or potential. But our internal discourse is often much more critical, even self-destructive, and we use words that we wouldn't tolerate if they came from somebody else. As I recently read on a forum: "People say it's a jungle out there, but the real jungle is between their ears!"

Ask yourself this question: is your internal dialog compassionate and encouraging or are you critical and skeptical? Would you say the same thing to one of your friends?

So this tip is quite simple: when you talk to yourself don't use a tone or words that you wouldn't use to your best friend. What would you say to your best friend if she was in your shoes? "You're a failure. You are going to sound ridiculous and everybody will laugh at you!"?

This chapter is undoubtedly one of the most important in the book. Every time an opportunity for speaking appears on the horizon (interview, oral, presentation), as the date approaches, fear will come to haunt you. When it knocks on the door, don't let it in: use these six tips.

I WISH I HAD KNOWN THAT THE WORD 'FAILURE' DOESN'T EXIST. EVEN BAD EXPERIENCES ARE THE STEPPING STONES TO SUCCESS

By now you have found the necessary motivation to get going; you have made your resolutions and fixed your objectives. You have learnt to replace your fears by more constructive thoughts and you have taken your first concrete steps.

And now, obviously, things begin to get difficult and the initial results are not what you expected. You will notice that I **talk about results and not failures, which makes all the difference.**

Don't be disappointed by these results because:

In the first place, you should congratulate yourself on having put your intentions into practice. Remember, in order to be proud of yourself you should do things of which you are proud. In daring to begin and facing up to situations that you avoided up till now, you have shown your courage. As Tony Robbins said:

> No matter how many mistakes you make or how slow you progress, you are still way ahead of everyone who isn't trying.

These experiences will help you to progress. You are just starting your learning process, which makes you a novice. A novice skier will fall head over heels, a greenhorn juggler will drop his clubs, a rookie golfer will miss the ball. Until one day, by practicing and persevering, they will get into the swing of it, making the gestures automatically and confidently. Just as you will soon do in speaking situations. The most important thing is to learn from experience. What went well; what went less well? Why? How did you prepare yourself? Would it have been useful to have announced that you stutter? Nowadays, when a situation gets out of hand, I try to analyze it rather than to go in for self-punishment. As Churchill, yet another famous stutterer, said:

Success consists of going from failure to failure without loss of enthusiasm.

Just as you will be proud of having tried rather than having avoided the situation, you will also learn more about yourself, discovering skills you didn't even suspect you had. The strength of a man or a woman is measured not in terms of their misadventures but by their ability to pick themselves up again.

Before she became world famous and one of the richest women in the United Kingdom, **J K Rowling, the best-selling author of Harry Potter**, was an unemployed single mother with a young child, struggling to make ends meet. Speaking at Harvard University, this is what she said to students about setbacks:[18]

> Some failure in life is inevitable. It is impossible to live without failing at something, unless you live so cautiously that you might as well not have lived at all - in which case, you fail by default. (...) Failure taught me things about myself that I could have learned no other way. I discovered that I had a strong will, and

---

[18] http://news.harvard.edu/gazette/story/2008/06/text-of-j-k-rowling-speech/

more discipline than I had suspected; I also found out that I had friends whose value was truly above the price of rubies.

In the end, your strategy will pay back. Aim for long-term results rather than quick and easy victories. Something that seems impossible in the short term can be achievable in the long-term if you persist.

Everything you have learnt, you have learnt like this. Would you stop teaching your daughter to walk or ride a bicycle because she has fallen repeatedly? No, of course not, you would have to be mad! As for yourself, you have decided to break an enormous rock in the middle of the path. At the beginning, you have the impression that your hammer is making no impression. You continue hitting it twice, ten times, twenty times but the rock is still intact. Were the blows a waste of time? Should you give up? No! Because on the fiftieth blow - or perhaps even on the twenty-first - the rock will explode. Was it the last blow that pulverized it? **Of course not. It was the sum of all those previous blows which had seemed so ineffective.** Your efforts will not be in vain.

I WISH I HAD KNOWN THAT THERE ARE NO DIFFICULTIES, ONLY OPPORTUNITIES

Churchill sums up the importance of a positive attitude:

The pessimist sees difficulty in every opportunity. The optimist sees the opportunity in every difficulty.

Nevertheless, I should to be frank with you. Be warned: your progress won't be linear, like a ladder which you climb one rung after another. Sometimes you will slip and fall down several rungs to find yourself back near the bottom. **You really need to prepare yourself for the 'chutes' in your personal game of 'chutes and ladders', because they are disturbingly frequent.** Changing thoughts and behavior requires a long and sometimes slow reprogramming. And one of the difficulties in speech therapy is that bad habits can come back very quickly even though you thought you had eliminated them definitively. It is important to prepare yourself for what I am now going to describe as it happens frequently. You have already learnt how to face up to the Wicked Witch of Fear; now you must prepare yourself to meet her sneering friend, Relapse.

Here's what might happen. After several failed attempts, you finally find a method or a therapy which suits you. You have successfully completed your speech therapy sessions or your course and you have achieved fluency. You take part in conversations and you interact with strangers. Your parents and your friends can't believe it. You are transformed and you feel powerful and invincible for the first time. Another novelty: you take pleasure in communicating. Words come easily and you think that finally something has just clicked. You believe that you have overcome your stutter and that you have, at long last, found the means of expressing yourself. And you understand how you have done it.

The situation lasts several days, perhaps several weeks. And then some difficulties start to reappear; the motor misfires from time to time. At first, it is just a slight irritation but enough for doubts to penetrate your mind. You lose confidence in the method you have learnt, you are less assiduous in applying it, and your former reflexes resurface. You avoid a few words or an opportunity to speak. A slight whiff of stress and wham! You're back where you were. A story that you couldn't tell, a failed undertaking or a missed telephone call; you feel as if you have been hit by a tidal wave, and have washed up at your starting point. It is just all too much. You are *so* disappointed. The euphoric heights you reached only a few days previously are left behind in your rapid descent. Your fluency has disappeared. Where the heck has it gone?

Don't panic; it's normal!

Many people who stutter believe that fluency acquired in therapy sessions or on an intensive course will last without continued work. Relapse is a crucial problem encountered in the treatment of stuttering. Some therapists emphasize, slightly provocatively, that: "It isn't very complicated to make a stutterer talk fluently; the problem is to maintain that fluency".

Learning a technique or setting oneself an objective (for example, I will stop hiding my stuttering and using subterfuges) is quickly done; it takes much longer to change one's thoughts and behavior.

Stuttering has been a part of you for many years. It won't disappear in a few weeks or even in a few months. So you must be prepared for relapses if you wish to deal with it without being upset. Make your setback into a positive experience: why did I mess up, what did I or didn't I do, what was I thinking about, how did I react, did I use the techniques I have learnt, and if not, why not?

A few years ago, I wanted to learn how to juggle with three balls. It took me weeks and hundreds, perhaps thousands, of attempts. I was often irritated. If I had given up and put my juggling balls away, I wouldn't now be able to juggle. So what, you might say. To some extent you are right, but persevering in this futile learning process improved my self-confidence. At first I was really hopeless. The balls went everywhere. At one time I even thought that I wasn't physically capable of accomplishing this exercise and that I would never succeed (does that remind you of anything?). And then, one day, I managed five seconds of juggling without dropping the balls, then a little longer... Little by little I progressed. I dropped the balls less and less frequently, until the day came when the gestures started to become automatic.

Now, thanks to this little trick, I have reinforced my children's belief that I am a living god: all I have to do is to carelessly juggle three oranges from time to time. And watch their eyes light up.

So, when you have found a method which works for you or made a resolution, don't get discouraged: persevere, tell yourself that relapses are completely normal and don't mean you are a failure. They are nothing to do with you, your personality or your performance. They are simply a logical part of every learning process.

The problem is that we have a tendency to focus on what went wrong, forgetting our previous victories. Charles Van Riper understood this, reminding speech therapists that stutterers "minimize their successes" and "maximize their setbacks". And this way of thinking isn't limited to people who stutter. As the French actor Pierre Arditti explained in an interview:

A compliment gives me three minutes of pleasure but I ruminate over a bad review for three days.

So it is important to build on your past successes and all those things you have already learnt. Rejoice in the achievements in your life, however trivial they are.

As I suggested in the previous chapter, keeping a diary will enable you to keep your setbacks in perspective so that they don't make you forget your successes. Lazarus and Fay, the authors of *I Can if I Want To*[19] think that patients should record their triumphs because it reinforces them. They go as far as to predict "no notebook, no change". Patients are encouraged to keep a journal and to write down their successes, whether they were expected or not. Many teenagers have reported that regularly reading out loud what they have written, in particular when they were feeling insecure or surrounded by negative thoughts, turned out to be very useful.

It is important to note your triumphs so as not to forget them and stop them being buried under a heap

---

[19] *I can if I want to* by Arnold Lazarus and Allen Fay – FMC Books.

of negative experiences. You should reread them when you are feeling insecure so as to remember that:

you aren't a complete failure,

you have been able to speak successfully.

And above all, you now know that fluency is possible and not merely a pipedream. It is within your grasp; you have held it in your hand. When writing about your achievements, remember to note your state of mind and how the triumph came about, reviewing the events of the days which led up to it. Your diary is like a store cupboard where you keep the ingredients of your successful recipe.

In the next chapter, I would like to share another important lesson on this theme.

I WISH I HAD KNOWN THAT

STUTTERING IS NOT A FAILURE AND

FLUENCY IS NOT A SUCCESS

Recognizing this is essential for your progress. You must stop analyzing your success in speaking by your level of fluency or your stuttering.

Perfect fluency is a fantasy. Watch other people and listen carefully. You will notice that everybody trips up, repeats things, hesitates, uses fillers (well, ugh, in fact, etc.). Often they don't even notice because they aren't trying to avoid them and also because communication is composed of a multitude of other elements: enthusiasm, smiling, gestures, listening, and so on. Therefore, keep in mind that you are practicing so that you can talk when you like and take pleasure in communicating rather than trying to be perfectly fluent.

Success, the reward for all your efforts, is about being able to say what you want, when you want, to whom you want. And the number of times you stutter isn't important. Most people consider themselves 'cured' when: firstly they have rid themselves of their fear of stuttering, secondly they stop avoiding speaking situations and thirdly their oral communication is completely satisfactory in most situations. They report that they still sometimes trip over words but the big difference is that they no longer consider it the end of the world. They have rediscovered their self-esteem and confidence in speaking. This is what Charlie says on my blog:

For someone who stutters, the objective is to be capable of saying the words without thinking about stuttering. I consider myself to be 100% fluent despite the fact that I stick occasionally. I say this because I am no longer afraid of speaking in public. I can confront any of the situations which previously used to terrorize me. I no longer need to substitute words. I know that I can speak fluently. When I speak the words come easily and I don't think about stuttering. On the rare occasions when it resurfaces, I use my techniques to get over it and push it aside. Having confidence in my speaking has enriched my life immensely.

It is the same for Anna,[20] who doesn't think in terms of stuttering anymore. She explains:

I feel that stuttering has lost its significance for me. It is a very strange feeling, like when you meet an old boyfriend from your schooldays. You are no longer affected by whatever it was that used to move you. Even when I see myself stuttering on a video, I am unaffected. When I speak, I don't pay any more attention to tripping over my words than I would if I tripped whilst walking.

So stop thinking in terms of fluency or stuttering and follow John Harrison's wise advice:

The only things you need to ask yourself are: (1) Did I keep to my intentions? and (2) did I have fun?

If you succeeded in one of the two, you have won. If you succeed in both then, as they say in baseball, you hit a home run.

---

[20] Anna's story is featured on www.masteringstuttering.com. She entitled it "Befrieding my monster was the key to recovery". Not to be missed.

I WISH I HAD KNOWN THAT "WE ARE WHAT WE REPEATEDLY DO. EXCELLENCE, THEN, IS NOT AN ACT, BUT A HABIT." – ARISTOTLE

That's the real message of the last chapter: changing may take some time because stuttering has been directing your thoughts and actions for years.

How long, you may well ask? My reply is: as long as you want! If you practice using the telephone three times a day your rate of progress will be ninety times quicker than if you only do it once a month.

However, there is a more precise and more scientific answer to the question. Phillippa Lally and her colleagues at University College London studied 96 people[21] who had decided to change their lives for the better by resolving, for example, to eat a fruit at

---

[21] How habits are formed : Modelling habit formation in the real world – Phillippa Lally - *European Journal of Social Psychology* 16 July 2009

breakfast time or going jogging for 15 minutes a day. The conclusions confirm what we already know. On the one hand, the more regularly you repeat an action the more it tends to become automatic. And on the other hand, this doesn't happen in three days. But what is particularly interesting is that the study has measured the average time needed to form a habit. And this time is (drum roll... wait for it...) 66 days!

Of course this is an average and everything depends on your motivation and the complexity of the behavior you wish to develop. However, if you have decided to stop avoiding words you are afraid of, or to keep eye contact when you stutter, now you know that you need to continue for at least two months before getting discouraged and saying that it doesn't work.

So, practice every day. Let's stay with the example of the telephone. Reply to newspaper adverts, arrange appointments, cancel them, phone free numbers for information. When you are at home, try to be the person who picks up the phone. The aim is to reduce your anxiety, to practice the advice given above and to learn from making calls. Progress comes from repeated practice; there is no more effective way.

A few years ago I preferred to walk along corridors and climb stairs rather than to call a colleague. At home, I asked my wife to make certain calls for me. Nowadays, I pick up the phone without even thinking, simply because it has become a habit, an everyday act which I no longer fear, as banal and normal as getting on a bicycle and pushing on the pedals. If I had continued with avoiding, if I hadn't practiced every day, I wouldn't be where I am today.

A constant determination to tackle what we fear also works very well for the words and sounds we dread. **The simplest and undoubtedly the most effective strategy is 'machine gunning'.** The aim is to confront the feared sound, again and again, until it loses any negative connotation. By tackling the sound head-on, by showing that you are not even a teeny-weeny bit afraid, you will flatten the obstacle in your path, to the point that when you pass over it you won't feel the least jolt or apprehension.

One technique which desensitizes you from fear of stuttering is called 'voluntary stuttering'. How mad can you get? you might say. Indeed, at first glance, it seems idiotic to practice stuttering when you are looking for the exact opposite. Nevertheless, some people cite this technique as one of those which most helped in their treatment: one of Lon L. Emerick's patients found success through this method:[22]

> The more you stutter on purpose, the less you hold back; and the less you hold back, the less you stutter. We once worked with a young exchange student who almost completely extinguished her stuttering in one week by doing negative practice. We were enmeshed in doctoral examinations so we gave her a handcounter and told her: 'There are 100,000 people living in Lansing; see how many you can talk to and show your stuttering.' When I saw her seven days later she was haggard and worn but grinning broadly and not stuttering. Having taken us literally she had worked around the clock. Incredibly she had confronted 947 listeners! And she was totally unable to stutter involuntarily.

Personally, I particularly dreaded having to introduce myself, from fear of blocking on my name and hearing an ironic: "You've forgotten your own name?" So I practiced incessantly in front of a mirror, when walking, when driving: "Hello, I'm Laurent

---

[22] American therapist who stuttered himself. He is one of the authors of *Advice to Those Who Stutter*.

Lagarde". The only problem is that I talk in my sleep and my wife was woken up more than once in the middle of the night by an impeccable though rather loud: "Hello, I'm Laurent Lagarde!"

This intensive method was inspired by a conversation I had with a former stutterer a few years ago. After months of good fluency, he had suddenly started to fear words beginning with a certain sound.

'So what did you do?' I asked him.

He replied: 'I killed it. Simply killed it. I spent an entire day on the street asking for whatever came into my head as long as it began with this sound. I must have done it more than 150 times. At the end of the day the fear had disappeared.'

Of course, perhaps it won't work for everyone but one thing is certain: nobody can say that it hasn't worked unless they have tried it more than 150 times... and 66 days.

I WISH I HAD KNOWN THAT SOME OF THE BEST SPEAKERS IN THE WORLD STUTTER

Your mouth can spit venom, or it can mend a broken soul. Words are power. Words can be your power. You can change a life, inspire a nation, make this world a beautiful place.

Who would believe that these words were uttered by someone who stutters? And that he has become a world champion in his discipline: public speaking? Nevertheless it's true. Mohammed Qahtani from Saudi Arabia won the Toastmasters'[23] eloquence competition in 2015 beating 30,000 participants from 100 countries over a period of six months. The talk that he gave in the final was "The power of words".

---

[23] The story of the Toastmasters' clubs begins in 1905, with the initiative of Ralph C. Smedley, who was the director of a YMCA centre in Illinois at that time. Noticing that some of the young men who came to the centre had great difficulty in speaking in public or participating in meetings, he had the idea of creating clubs where they could learn how to express themselves. As a result, today there are nearly 16,000 Toastmasters' clubs in 142 countries. For more information see https://www.toastmasters.org/

As a child, Mohammed was mocked for his pronounced stutter. At the prize-giving ceremony he urged the people in the audience to face up to their fears. "I used to be the laughing stock at school, but look at me now. If this can happen to me, imagine what could happen to you."[24]

Perhaps you think this fairy tale is exceptional and has nothing to do with you. You're wrong. Innumerable stutterers who used to panic when faced with an opportunity to speak now bathe in the pleasure of audience applause.

I have already mentioned John Moore, a presenter who stutters, and Alan Badmington in previous chapters. They have both overcome their pronounced stutter and are now invited to give talks all over the world. For them, speaking in public has become a source of immense pleasure; they are applauded wherever they go.

After hearing Alan speak at an American speech therapists' congress, one participant, Brian, came back full of enthusiasm.

---

[24] https://mediacenter.toastmasters.org/2015-08-17-Saudi-Arabian-engineer-wins-Toastmasters-2015-World-Championship-of-Public-Speaking

He was amazing: he had a standing ovation after his talk on his personal development and the role self-help groups had had in his journey towards fluency. For those professional speech therapists present it was a powerful message. Being myself a speech therapist who stutters, I too was greatly impressed. In short, we must widen our comfort zone by challenging ourselves, going beyond our constricting beliefs. That talk will always stay with me. Alan, you are a real gift for everyone who stutters.

John and Alan are not isolated cases. Like Mohammed, Anna also decided to join a Toastmasters club to practice public speaking. Then she started participating in competitions, and winning them! One of her successes was to carry off the first prize in the "District Humorous Speech Contest" where she was up against champions from other local clubs. She had to speak in front of an audience and five judges; worse, the time was limited. "The best thing about it for me was the way the public reacted," she said. "Both the experience and the reaction were incredible."

Geneviève, vice-president of the Association des Bègues du Canada [Canadian Stutterers Association] has also tried the Toastmasters' experience.

On that occasion, I had to do four talks. The stress decreased each time. I soon realized that the confidence I gained during those evenings could be transferred easily to everyday situations. I was particularly surprised when I had to do a training course for work that my heart didn't race when it came to my turn to talk. I was delighted by my new-found assurance.[25]

As for Anne-Fleur, for a long time she lived in fear of stuttering and suffered in consequence.

At school, I had to swallow everything. I was called a 'broken record'. I was openly mocked. The worst thing was when kids imitated me by making grotesque noises. I had the impression that my life consisted of policing everything I said. It was like having a bomb where my mouth should have been.

One day she decided she had had enough "of being reduced to the rank of a stutterer and finding my tongue tied in knots every time I wanted to speak". So she took her courage in both hands and started participating in Model United Nations (MUN) conferences at her university. These conferences are

---

[25] https://monjolibegaiement.wordpress.com/2017/03/06/les-toastmasters-ou-lart-de-la-desensibilisation/

intended to simulate the workings of the United Nations, giving students the opportunity to take on the role of diplomats and debate international political issues according to UN rules.

For Anne-Fleur it was a long haul, but enriching. She learnt to overcome her fears and became a champion orator and then a coach for international diplomatic competitions.

I learnt from that experience that **there is no such thing as a little challenge**. And, more importantly, even if we are unaware of it we all have what is necessary to succeed.[26]

Anne-Fleur is right: it isn't a small challenge. Fear of public speaking is actually the most common of all phobias: 75% of people are afraid of speaking in front of an audience. It even has a name: glossophobia.

Unsurprisingly then, I was a glossophobe for many years. Panicking at the thought at having to speak in public was a part of my life. The very idea triggered overpowering physical symptoms. This is what I wrote in my diary in 2004:

---

[26] http://www.madmoizelle.com/begue-concours-eloquence-762139

I'm sure I'm going to muck it up. I'm going to butt head first against a word or a phrase. It will make the other participants ill-at-ease, they will get annoyed, judge me... And when that happens I will instantly and automatically enter stuttering mode.

Something in my sternum will crush my chest and block my trachea. It's like diving into the sea holding my breath. My brain lacks oxygen. I am a prisoner of fear. I am in a tiny room where fear is king. I am dizzy, I am only half breathing, my lungs cannot expand enough. I have a slight headache, the uncomfortable feeling that the top half of my body is overheating, the impression that my lungs are only half full.

Then the block arrives: a flap shuts at the top of my trachea and the air no longer circulates. I can neither breathe in nor breathe out. At its worst, I feel a very strange kind of emptiness, like a transient inability to register my surroundings, where the only thing that matters is to get that word or phrase out...

Rereading these words, a powerful image comes back to me: the opening scene of the film 'The King's Speech' when Colin Firth, playing the future King George VI, has to speak before a stadium full of people. It is a measure of Firth's skill that he manages to convey the distress suffered by people who stutter when faced with such a situation.

And then one day, like Anne-Fleur, I decided that things couldn't continue like that. I had to do a presentation for a small audience and the president of the bank where I worked. I was so sick at the thought of it that I said to my wife that I was going to ask my boss to replace me. It would be best to accept that I wasn't made for it and leave someone else to take my place. But I realized that I would be much worse if I avoided the problem. I would undermine my confidence in my ability to speak and the next time I needed to do it the stress would certainly be worse. So I said to myself that I must defuse the situation: most of the people who would be present knew that I sometimes had elocution problems. I should accept it, even if it meant that I had to joke about it or take a break if it really came to the worst.

As a result I decided to face up to the situation and do everything possible to make things go smoothly. That was only the beginning of a great adventure. It hasn't always been easy, but that decision was the basis of the enormous progress I have since made.

Working on public speaking has been a giant leap in my walk on the lunar surface of stuttering.

Nowadays I regularly do presentations at work and I have also been invited to lecture at conferences on stuttering. Previously, faced with these gatherings – in places such as amphitheaters and congress halls – I would have run a mile.

How do I prepare and manage these situations? As you will see it is simply the practical application of everything we have learnt in the previous chapters.

Here are nine tips on public speaking for people who stutter

1. Prepare yourself.

Preparation is essential. It is the basis of my self-confidence. It is stupid to add to the stress of the presentation by being badly prepared. The more you plan ahead, the less nervous you are. It is also a form of respect for your audience. In fact, you should be thinking of them in the first place when you are preparing your presentation. Ask yourself, what can I give them? Think about how your talk can benefit them.

Changing your viewpoint like this – going from 'me' to 'them' – is essential. Because we are obsessed by our stuttering, all too often we are egocentric, which feeds our fear. Will they like *me*? Will they find *my* talk interesting? Will they laugh at *me*? Will I lose *my* thread? Will they think *I* am good? Stop thinking about yourself! Stop going round in circles! This way of thinking stops you moving forward! Try instead to concentrate on your audience and ask yourself this question: how can I help my listeners? How can I be useful? This is the way to relegate ideas about your performance to the dressing room along with the pressure which accompanies them. Do not try to impress your audience. Instead try to emphasize sharing information and sharing ideas.

When I step onto the stage I am not there to perform, nor to show that I am a nice guy. I am there because I think I can be of use to my listeners. What matters is to help, not to shine.

I was recently invited to speak to 180 speech therapists. So I said to myself, have I got an answer to the kind of questions they ask themselves? And there was my subject, a subject which comes up regularly and which is a mystery to speech therapists: why does my patient's stuttering often disappear after a few sessions only to come back again as soon as she leaves my office? How can I succeed in helping her to transfer this fluidity to 'real' life?

The conference went very well, not because I was a great performer, a master of the spoken word, but because I had aroused their curiosity and shown that I was interested in them, that I hadn't come to spew out a presentation I had already given a hundred times before. From then on, they were prepared to listen to me, with or without stuttering. If you approach the experience in the spirit of helping and enlightening, rather than trying to sell yourself or to make yourself popular, your listeners will feel it and hold out a welcoming hand.

In general, once I have thought these things through I compose my presentation, by which I mean the answer to the question, dividing my talk into sections: introduction, point no. 1, point no. 2, point no. 3, conclusion. Then I write the main ideas down on paper. These are checklists that I will use for brushing up my talk. It is also reassuring to have them to hand during the event. The aim is to avoid worrying about what I will say, to eliminate the fear of forgetting and to be able to rely on them if I am really too stressed. These cards are my lifeline; I can let go of it if I feel relaxed. I don't write whole sentences, just scribble a few key words. Unless you're very talented, there's nothing more boring than a text read out loud or recited from memory. I allow myself just one exception to this rule: I commit the first few sentences of my introduction to memory because it is then, during those first thirty seconds, that the tension is at its height. Committing the introduction to memory means you can keep cool.

I remember my first speech in an amphitheater; it was for work. When the fateful moment arrived, I walked towards the lectern as if I was going to be burned at the stake. When it came to pronouncing the first word, a great wave of stress washed over me and the first sentences were hard going. The words didn't come; I felt I was tearing them from my throat one by one. However, I managed to keep to my text even though I had the impression of plowing through it. Astonishingly, a colleague who was present in the room told me that he hadn't seen it that way. I had given him the impression of concentrating hard on my subject, which had captured his attention.

I am convinced that this preparatory work, so often neglected, is our strength. So many people step onto the stage without having really prepared themselves, without having adapted themselves to their listeners. With the result that their presentations are too long, wandering, confused or abstruse. You listeners will be grateful that you haven't fallen into these traps.

2. Be concise: less is better!

When I started doing presentations, I made sure that they lasted the shortest time possible. I wanted to get the ordeal over as quickly as possible. So I resolved to be as concise as possible, to avoid diluting my subject, going straight to the essentials. Over the years, I have discovered that this objective, which was initially imposed by my stuttering, was a strength and made me stand out from other speakers.

When you present a subject, especially something you are passionate about, you tend to want to say everything you know, incorporating all those funny anecdotes you have collected. That's a mistake. You risk drowning your listeners in a flood of information and boring them with your long analysis. Being concise will help you to clarify your ideas and make your message clear. It will help you select the most pertinent details, those which need to be remembered.

Don't try to find a place for all those formidable things you have to say. You don't need to display all the knowledge you have acquired on the subject. Chose two or three ideas that you want to pass on. Less is better.

Being concise is a strength. Many people water down their talk and get lost in the details, so that someone who goes straight to the point – and sticks to the allotted time – is appreciated. Especially when ten speakers come onto the stage one after another!

3. Practice

Having written my text and prepared my index cards, I practice my presentation by reading it out loud. I go through it literally dozens of times, day after day, all of which enables me to make corrections, cut waffle and join the different sections together. By the time the big day arrives I almost know my text and the order of presentation off by heart, which gives me the vital confidence I need.

I have recently discovered an original way of practicing. The Japanese writer Haruki Marukami, author of the *1Q84* trilogy, gets invited to give lectures around the world. He is also a running fanatic. In his book *What I Talk About When I Talk About Running* he explains that he practices his presentations while running. I was intrigued, so I tried this unusual method and can confirm that it is very effective. New ideas emerge as I move along, I learn to manage my breathing, to speak more slowly and to insert pauses. It even helps my running because my mind is busy and doesn't have the time to think about my body; the time passes much more quickly and I run for longer. It could well be that the people I meet have doubts about my sanity, but I don't care.

I also advise practicing in front of a friend. This simulates the situation of being in front of an audience and you will get feedback on how you are doing. It is another rung on the ladder to success. Of course, you can do this with your therapist as did Geneviève. She had an appointment with her speech therapist just before doing a presentation for her literature class:

I took the opportunity to practice my talk with her. It came at just the right time. We had just finished reviewing techniques and had reached the stage where I had to use them in 'real-life' situations. So I applied the techniques to practicing the presentation. It did me so much good! We even went out into the waiting room because I wanted to avoid the comfort of her office. My therapist was really pleased that I had taken the initiative. It was also very effective; being in the waiting room made me feel more like I was in class.

Another stutterer, Betty, had to give a talk at the AGM of the bank where she works in front of clients and under the eagle eye of her bosses. She too recognizes the benefits of practice:

I rehearsed my text night and day. In my car, with my speech therapist, with my husband and my son, at bedtime. I knew what I was going to say and how to say it.

Betty has summarized the benefits of preparation and rehearsing perfectly: you know what you are going to say and how you are going to say it. By this point you have already done ninety percent of the work necessary for a successful presentation. The only thing left is to work on your state of mind on the big day.

4. Prepare to stutter.

Your attitude to the experience is crucial. The previous steps have neutralized any fear about what you are going to say. So there 'only' remains the fear of stuttering.

To get rid of this, I needed to change my viewpoint. This is the stage of 'acceptance' which I mentioned at the beginning of the book: understanding that stuttering is not a fault and not my fault. I accepted that I may stutter but that it is a part of me and that I am not responsible for it. Stuttering makes me different and I accept this state of affairs, neither proud nor ashamed. I am someone who stutters and I may stutter from time to time during my presentation but I won't consider it a catastrophe. I have replaced "Oh my God, above all I mustn't stutter" with "Perhaps I will stutter. What should I do if it happens?" Here too, you need to forget any idea of performance or perfection. Ruling out stuttering is the best way of putting yourself under enormous pressure.

It seems to me that this is the point for a little revision. What is the best way of eliminating this fear of stuttering, this fear of being exposed? Do you remember? Go back a few pages... Yes! Tell people that you stutter. Pull the cat out of the bag. John Moore has no quandaries about it:

> We invest so much mental and physical energy avoiding stuttering that it increases our anxiety when we speak. Which generates the stuttering. I have discovered that it is very useful to mention my stutter at the beginning of my presentations. Not only does this disarm the public but also it gives me as a person who stutters the liberty to stutter without shame.

Silvano, who was the last of a long series of speakers at a briefing, started his talk as follows:

> I have some good news and some bad news. The good news is that I am the last speaker, the bad news is that I am a stutterer ... so who knows how long it's gonna take!

In fact stuttering gives us an advantage over other mortals! We have an excuse for being stressed!

You also need to work on the question of what to do if you stutter knowing that, thanks to your warning, your public won't be surprised. You can make a joke of it, try a fluency technique to get over the block, pause, etc. It's up to you to find the method that suits you. Here too, the fact that you are prepared for the eventuality will allow you to tackle it confidently. And your confidence will grow with each new presentation.

But above all do not worry about the times when you stutter: effective communication isn't a question of fluency. Take for example Russ Hicks, who has won numerous Toastmasters' competitions.

> I stutter all the time! It's just that the judges didn't care. They thought I communicated more effectively than the rest of the contestants. I've often wondered if there wasn't some level of minimum fluency that makes public speaking worthwhile. My initial reaction is yes, there is. But just when I try to define it, a severe stutterer comes along and proves me wrong.

5. Work on your posture

As with every form of communication, a presentation or an analysis isn't just a question of the spoken word. Your behavior and your gestures are also part of the message. It is important to keep this in mind, especially as one's posture has a direct influence on one's thoughts. To understand this, nothing better than to try this little exercise proposed by Keith Boss, a fellow stutterer.

Stand tall, shoulders back, chin up, very big smile. What are you thinking?

Now slump down, shoulders hunched, face hanging down, frowning and almost crying. What different things are you thinking?

The importance of posture is underlined by orators who stutter, John Moore amongst them:

I have become successful by focusing more on my bearing and my self-assurance on stage than on the words I use. Keeping visual contact with my audience, adopting a good posture and using gestures gives me greater fluency on stage.

Anne-Fleur also stresses this point when she is coaching:

> I teach students – above all the girls – to take possession of the debate both **physically and verbally**. To stand firmly on their feet, to use body language to show their ownership, to fully inhabit the space, a space which we women have been taught to reduce since our childhood. Stop being small, cute and discreet!

So, when it is my turn to speak, I take a little time before starting. I raise my shoulders, smile and look at the audience. This is my way of taking possession of the space and creating a calm, reassuring atmosphere, conductive to relaxation and listening. It is also a way of banishing negative thoughts and stopping me rushing into things.

6. Smile!

I particularly remember one of my first successful speeches at work. I had to present the results of a marketing strategy to colleagues from throughout France. I was already on the stage a few minutes before my turn, waiting for the previous speaker to finish. I scanned the room and noticed a man in the front row. His expressionless face showed that he was very bored. His black eyes were staring at me. At first I said to myself: "Oh! Oh! That guy doesn't look a bundle of laughs. He's going to judge me and he won't be at all forgiving..." Guess what I did to counter my negative instincts. I smiled at him... And the result was immediate: he smiled back! So I then smiled at everybody whose eye I caught and they all smiled back. Even before I had started I already had a room full of friends!

Smile! Smile when you approach the lectern, smile before starting, smile when you are speaking and smile when you finish. Smile when you leave the stage. Smile.

It isn't just about making contact with the audience. Psychologists from the University of Kansas[27] have proved that a smile, even if forced, can reduce stress. The heart rate of those who smiled during the experiment was lower than that of those who didn't. So, once again, think about your audience. It is definitely more enjoyable listening to someone who smiles.

---

[27] https://www.psychologicalscience.org/news/releases/smiling-facilitates-stress-recovery.html

If you have a block, continue to smile to show that it isn't important, just a little interruption. Some people even claim that it is impossible to smile and stutter at the same time. You can try it. In fact, I bet you are already trying it. ☺

7. Make them laugh!

Humor and a making fun of oneself – within limits – are precious allies, and effective too.

They came in handy on the day I've been talking about. I was still a little tense when it came to my turn despite all the new smiling friends I had just made. So, hoping to defuse the situation a little, when I came to my second slide I tested my first witticism. I was the second last speaker of the day and everybody was somewhat tired. This is what I said: "This slide is very interesting. In fact, it is the most interesting one in my presentation. The rest are not great, so I suggest that you look at it carefully. Afterwards you can go back to sleep!" Everybody laughed; the connection was made. From that moment on I let myself go and really took pleasure in what I was doing. I was no longer worried and spoke in a more natural and relaxed way. I even drew some applause.

Mohammed Qahtani, the word champion mentioned above, started his presentation by pretending to light a cigarette. When the audience reacted he started defending the tobacco industry before finally revealing that all the figures and studies he had just cited were entirely made up, which made them laugh. "When you get an audience laughing, you've got them on your side. Don't forget that an audience is waiting to be entertained." One day, a member of his Toastmasters' club said to him: "Some people's strength is in their choice of words. Others rely on their voice or their behavior. Your strength is your humor. Use it." And that is exactly what helped him win despite competing with people who did not stutter.

8. Slow down

The symptoms of stress are increasing heart rate and – often – talking faster. So it is vital to concentrate on slowing down. Indeed, many therapies for people who stutter are based on this principle. Having learnt your first sentences by heart will be a great help. You will thus eliminate the stress of improvisation; relying on words you know will keep you confidently on track. It is important to have practiced them by talking slowly. You will start at the right speed and arrive at your goal still fresh.

I have come across some speakers who are passionate about their subject and who start out brilliantly. But after a few minutes they start to drown their listeners in a torrent of words recited at top speed without the least interruption. Don't fall into that trap.

I'll let you into a little secret. You don't need to adopt the listless phrasing of a tortoise (imagine how they would talk!). What you need is the art of the pause.

This subtle art, notably used by President Obama (watch the videos of his speeches and you will understand), is your best friend.

Pauses let you catch your breath, stop your tongue running away with itself, and keep your voice box in trim. As Alan Badmington says: "Pauses create a feeling of tranquility and calm composure. They contrast sharply with the confusion, nervousness and agitation to which I had become accustomed."

They allow you time to stay in contact with your listeners and to check that they have understood your propositions. You reduce the burden of the information you are sharing and thus give them the time to assimilate your words.

Pauses create tension (in a positive way): the wait encourages listening. Anne-Fleur teaches this technique to her students:

> I explain how to drop silences and pauses into their talks to kindle the audience's curiosity (because in a talk, speech may well be silver but silence is golden. It attracts attention, giving the words a golden setting).

To organize these pauses you need to divide your words into sequences. To do this, cut your sentences into phrases which make sense. It is much easier and less stressful to fix yourself the objective of pronouncing five words rather than twenty. This will also let you concentrate more on the articulation as well as the meaning of the words. When I started to apply this technique to public speaking it changed lots of things for me. Before, I stepped up to the lectern saying to myself: "My God, I'm going to have to talk for a quarter of an hour or half an hour". And the end of my torture seemed horribly far away. Now I can say to myself: "I am going to pay attention to making myself understood. My talk is a collection of beads which I am going to thread together calmly until I arrive at the end."

Having prepared your index cards and worked on being concise will help; your ideas are clear, you know that you have much information to share and that you have the time to pause and let your audience digest the important points. You will soon see that these short, clear phrases ram home your message and give it weight.

Don't think of your lecture as a chore to get finished, a race in which the only aim is to arrive at the finishing line. There is pleasure to be found along the way. Savor the moments together with your audience. Give them the time to understand and reflect on what you say.

9. Practice!

Speaking in public may seem an impossible goal to you. I can reassure you: every single one of those people I have quoted above felt the same.

Nevertheless, they managed it and now take immense pleasure in doing so. It is merely a learning process, acquiring skills and experience. As Russ Hicks says: "Public speaking is a learned art. Anyone can learn it, stutterer or not." The only thing you need to do is get started (remember: don't wait to be good before you start but start so you can be good) and practice.

In addition, we have the good luck, as people who stutter, of having associations that will welcome us. In the United States the National Stuttering Association[28] has more than 200 'chapters' as they are called. These are places where you will find an exceptional environment. An ideal place to practice, with other participants who will look on you with a sympathetic eye. At this point I would like to thank the Association Parole Bégaiement [French Stuttering Association] for inviting me to give my first public talks about my experiences. It was a great opportunity and enabled me to begin in a 'safe' environment before graduating to other challenges. For me, this was a first step in what became a progressive desensitization program – as mentioned above – allowing me to challenge my

---

[28] www.westutter.org

glossophobia. You only need to put your foot on the first rung of the ladder.

So, just do it!

I WISH I HAD KNOWN THAT STUTTERING DOESN'T STOP YOU FOLLOWING THE CAREER OF YOUR DREAMS, BE IT PHYSICIAN, SALESPERSON, ATTORNEY ETC.

As the last chapter has shown, we are all capable of doing things that seem impossible. This is something to keep in mind, particularly when you have projects that are dear to you. Don't let your stuttering limit you.

People often ask me questions about their choice of profession. I truly think you should not reject what seems an interesting career because you stutter. In my case, initially I chose jobs where I didn't need to open my mouth much, but finally my natural affinities pushed me towards marketing and then management, jobs where you often need to talk.

I'm not the only one. Despite continuing to stutter, Amy[29] has succeeded in becoming an actor and a singer. She has even worked in sales for several fashion labels. Her experience has taught her that fluency isn't necessary to communicate effectively at work.

> I regularly achieved the highest weekly sales in the team. As a child, I would never have dreamed this possible with a stutter!

I first met Sonia in 2010. At that time, she was participating in group discussion sessions for teenagers who stutter, organized by a speech therapist in Montpellier, France. She had already made considerable progress and told me that she wanted to study speech therapy.

We lost sight of each other until the day, three years later, when I received an email in which she said: "I am in my second year of studying speech therapy and I love it! I have truly found my vocation! I find the classes fascinating and enjoy learning."

---

[29] https://www.stammering.org/speaking-out/articles/job-talk

Since then she has obtained her diploma (passing easily) and realized her dream. And all that because she kept saying to herself: "don't let your stuttering stop you following the career you love!"

Patrick Brown's story is even more astonishing. The Canadian politician once mused: who would have thought that a kid that couldn't speak would now be leading a political party, where his job is to speak all day? He was talking about himself, of course, living proof that anything is possible and that you shouldn't abandon your dreams, whether you stutter or not.

There are some residual elements. There are some words that I'll trip over that are natural for others; that's a reminder of where I came from. But I don't feel uncomfortable at all anymore, I actually enjoy public speaking now and I might do it 10 times a day... At the time, it was a deep embarrassment but, in retrospect, I think moments of adversity build character and make you stronger, and I don't regret having to go through that. If you have to work harder, it makes you appreciate things more.[30]

In 2016 I was invited to the annual meeting of the Association des Bègues du Canada [Canadian Stutterers' Association for French-speakers] in Montreal. One of the wonderful local people I met was an attorney who stutters. Daniel was one of the speakers and talked about his own life. He explained how he had faced up to his personal demons one by one: telephone, Dictaphone, videoconference... and finally pleading before the court. He shared his conclusions:

Stuttering is inevitable. So you have to learn to live with it.

Don't try to fight it, or be afraid of it. Instead, tame it and learn to manage stressful situations. Practice makes perfect.

People are more interested in what I say than in how I say it. So I concentrate on controlling what I can control: the content (one of the keys to Daniel's success has been the great care he takes in preparing all his speaking engagements).

We have friends everywhere; nobody wants to see us fail.

I am so much more than a person who stutters!

Whatever your career, you have to speak.

In fact, I love speaking!

I have chosen Amy's, Sonia's, Patrick's and Daniel's stories because they show that anything is possible. Above all, I want you to accept one thing: fluent speaking is not a prerequisite for success. It is important to emphasize this point because I know that some people who stutter are discouraged rather than inspired by the role models presented to them. They are fed up to the teeth with those – often famous – people who have 'overcome' their stutter and talk about it with impressive fluency, without the slightest hint of hesitation, blocking or repetition. They find it difficult to identify with these 'stars', and may even have doubts about how much they stuttered in the past. For them perfect fluency remains a pipedream.

However, of all those people I have mentioned above, only Sonia has completely freed herself from her stuttering. **The others are not people who have overcome their stuttering in order to succeed but people who have succeeded whilst continuing to stutter.**

So get rid of all the unnecessary pressure that comes from thinking you must stop stuttering before doing certain studies or jobs. This is wrong, even for careers where communication is an important element. This is the lesson Amy has learnt from her time in sales, a job where one would think the spoken word was essential:

Although I have experienced high levels of anxiety, as well as frustration with my stutter and the painful feelings that can come with it, I have always been well respected and highly regarded by my managers, not least because of how they have perceived my communication skills. In my experience, effective communication and competency in one's job do not depend on fluency. I am very proud of this as a person who stutters, since selling involves high levels of social skills and communication.

This observation is not merely a figment of Amy's imagination. I was once invited by a colleague to a cocktail party given by his brother, the director of an advertising agency. The brother had invited all his clients and welcomed us all warmly. To my great surprise I discovered that he stuttered terribly. Really, it was one of the most severe stutters I have ever heard. I was astonished that he had managed to create such a successful agency. When he made his welcome speech everyone was delighted to listen to what he had to say. He stuttered enormously but it wasn't a problem for him or for his guests. I wouldn't even say that he acknowledged his stutter; it was of no importance to him. He smiled, he was enthusiastic and funny, and there was much applause. Afterwards, he passed from group to group and I had the impression that he had established a special relationship with his clients. He had no complexes, he wasn't hiding behind a mask, and his relaxed smile seemed infectious. Suddenly, his stuttering seemed to me to be a strength. It was the first time I had this sensation: that his stutter was part of his energy. It was his business card, what made him different. As he progressed, displaying his stutter for all to see, the faces around him lit up.

So don't make mastering your stutter into a precondition. And don't think that others will reject you because of it. Amy and Daniel haven't tried to hide their stutter and this has been accepted in their professional environment without difficulty. Amy explains that when she was being interviewed for a job in selling, she mentioned that she stuttered. Her future boss replied:

> The fact that you stutter makes no difference to me; my first impression of you was very positive. You have the right skills and experience for the role, are assertive, and an excellent communicator.

Sonia's case was a little different. Although she has now managed to control her stutter, when she was in her first year at university she had to undergo articulation and phonation tests with a speech therapist. Naturally she was very stressed but she decided to hide nothing and take responsibility for her choices.

> When she asked me if I had already been to see a speech therapist I didn't want to lie so I said "Yes, I was treated for stuttering. It's fine now' She appreciated my honesty and said "Our personal history often influences

our future". Then I had to do reading and counting exercises, and so on. I had one really tiny block but apart from that no stuttering at all during the tests. In her report the therapist said that everything was fine. I was so proud of myself.

Daniel is another person who has accepted his stutter. The Montreal legal association's magazine published a profile of him and it is very interesting to see how he is perceived.

He talks about his stutter frankly and with disarming ease. He speaks openly about it, defusing potentially embarrassing and tense situations by announcing it at the beginning. This is his way of reassuring people that his stutter is not because he is lackadaisical. He is ready to answer any questions or concerns they might have. His way of tackling stuttering head-on and never avoiding things which might worry him has always helped Daniel. It has enabled him to gain the respect of his peers as well as bringing hope to stutterers who feel they are restricted by their situation. Basically, Daniel doesn't give a damn about stuttering. He looks straight ahead, without fear and without regret, refusing to let his stuttering have a stranglehold over him.

Wonderful, isn't it? This experience really does confirm the golden rule: 'If we can live happily with our stutter, others will too'.

Who would have thought that a young man who stutters could one day become the vice-president of the United States? Well, that is what Joe Biden did. This is the lesson he wants to pass on:

> Your stutter doesn't define you. It has nothing to do with your intellectual capacities. In fact, it has nothing to do with anything which really counts... When you persevere in a fight, you will discover strengths that you didn't know you had, and that – I guarantee you – you will need one day.

Indeed, by following your own direction, one which you like, you will have to face up to speaking situations which you dread. You will learn to overcome them, which will have a positive effect on your ability to communicate. Following your vocation will give you the strength and enthusiasm needed to plan your future, to work and to persevere. Rather than asking yourself 'what negative impact will stuttering have on my chosen career?' ask instead 'what positive impact will my chosen career have on my stuttering?' If you choose a career where you have to talk, it will inevitably help you to progress in this area.

Amongst the things I thought I would never be able to do at the age of twenty were talking on the telephone, making conference calls, presenting a project, giving lectures... and I certainly wouldn't be able to do them today if I hadn't chosen a career that I like.

You must also take another factor into account. We often think about the risk involved in doing something, but have you thought about the risk of not doing it? Remember the vicious circle of avoidance. Rejecting a career which interests you is also taking a risk, that of frustration and low self-esteem.

Pam[31] was one of those people who didn't follow her vocation because she stuttered. Since then, she has done wonderful work on her blog to bring stuttering to the notice of the general public.

> I think a lot of my potential went unrealized. I let stuttering make decisions for me back then. I

---

[31] https://stutterrockstar.com/

always wanted to be a teacher. But I let stuttering, or more correctly, my fear of stuttering, make me steer clear of that. I settled for a career that I thought would involve less talking. (This of course turned out completely wrong!)

I wonder... can you relate to this? Did you ever feel you had poor self-esteem when it was actually unrealized potential? And have you let stuttering make decisions for you that you would choose differently if given a second chance?

The good news is that this second chance exists. Pam didn't become a teacher, but now she goes to schools regularly to explain to the children what stuttering is and how to react to it. She has received the Jefferson Award for her devotion and her public service.

Then again there is Lionel, whom I got to know via my blog. At forty he went back to study to be a speech therapist and has since been highly successful in his exams. There is also Alan Badmington, whom we have already met, who took up his lecturing career at the same age as many other retired people take up planting cabbages. (But who knows, maybe he plants cabbages as well. The two aren't incompatible.)

The website www.stammeringlaw.org.uk has a page[32] with many stories of people who stutter who have become actors, airline pilots, teachers, TV presenters, physicians, telephone advisors, driving instructors, attorneys, police officers, politicians and even priests![33]

There are no career limits and no age barrier if you want to realize your dreams. Your only limits are the ones which you set yourself.

---

[32] http://www.stammeringlaw.org.uk/employment/jobs.htm
[33] For more on priests, ministers and rabbis who stutter see the article 'God gave me my voice.' on www.goodbye-begaiement.fr.

I WISH I HAD KNOWN THAT I WAS NOT ALONE ... AND I WISH I HAD KNOWN THAT STUTTERING CAN OPEN A DOOR TO A WORLD OF WONDERFUL DISCOVERIES AND ENCOUNTERS

Now that you have decided to take steps to escape from the jaws of stuttering you will need help. It will be a thrilling but sometimes chaotic adventure and **it is easier if you travel in company.**

So far, you have undoubtedly felt alone. In my case, I had to wait twenty years before I could talk to someone who understood what I was feeling. When you stutter, you feel you are different and that nobody can understand your suffering and so you have a tendency to withdraw from society. You cut yourself off, start brooding on things, become frustrated, and so on. To the point where you sink into a real depression.

The solution, of course, is to break out of your shell, go out and meet people, communicate, and look for information on solutions. Unfortunately, it isn't always easy to confide in people you are close to; they have difficulty in understanding how much this 'minor aggravation' is ruining your life.

You have been dithering about coming out into the open and taking the first step towards other people. But that was before... Open the curtains, greet the sun, take a deep breath and prepare yourself to meet some delightful people. **Contact an association, go to a self-help group, get connected on social media. You will enjoy yourself and make friends.**

There is much more to people who stutter than their particular way of speaking, as you know when it comes to yourself. Stutterers are above all individuals in all their diversity, with different talents and qualities. You may well get to know them through their stuttering, but you will end up getting along with them for countless other reasons.

There are many ways of surrounding yourself with considerate people and escaping out of your isolation and into a constructive environment. For example, contact an association. Here are two to start with:

The Stuttering Foundation[34] has extensive information on topics such as prevention, early intervention, and therapy for stuttering as well as the latest information about basic research on stuttering. They provide a worldwide referral list of speech-language pathologists who specialize in stuttering; information about support groups in the U.S., Canada, and around the world. On The Stuttering Foundation Web, you will also find links to other websites that deal with stuttering, and information telling how to access listservs devoted to stuttering. It also has essays, stories, articles and case histories written by people who stutter as well as by clinicians.

The Canadian Stuttering Association[35] helps people who stutter and their families find reliable information and support. They organize information

---

[34] http://www.stutteringhelp.org/
[35] http://www.stutter.ca/

and social events and encourage support groups for people who stutter.

There are also self-help groups where you can meet regularly and talk in a relaxed way with other people who stutter. Typically, their program changes constantly: presentations, sharing experiences, debates, role-playing, theatrical sketches, etc. It is a bit like a house party for people who stutter. You will find a bit of everything there, beginning with what you bring yourself.

In addition, speech therapists organize group sessions for children and teenagers. These can help create strong links between the participants; some of the groups have given birth to remarkable projects. For example, a group of teenagers from Montpellier (France) presented the weather forecast on local television. And in Paris some others organized a survey asking passers-by what they knew about stuttering.

But if it seems premature to embark on this kind of thing, or you are not really a joining-in kind of person you can still meet people on the Internet. For some years now social media have been playing an important role in breaking down the isolation of people who stutter. The blogs and associations mentioned above have Facebook pages, including Goodbye Bégaiement,[36] of course.

Facebook is also an easy way of joining the British Stammering Association Support Group,[37] which has nearly 3000 members. There are some surprising discoveries to be made:

You are not alone: other people feel exactly as you do and have had identical experiences.

There are solutions. Many members of the association have tried various different therapies. For those that you find interesting you can benefit from the experiences of people who have gone before you. You can fill up your 'shopping cart' with the ones that suit you.

And above all, **you can express yourself**, which is to say do something which (perhaps) you have given up trying to do in 'real' life.

With the help of this magic potion of knowledge and experiences, you will find information to help you

---

[36] https://www.facebook.com/GoodbyeBegaiement
[37] https://www.facebook.com/groups/stammeringbsa/

better understand your stuttering, ideas for taming it and especially the support you need to bounce back and persevere when you are going through a bad patch. You will also have the satisfaction of being able to help others and the feeling that you have actively contributed to the 'fight' against stuttering.

David Shapiro is a renowned specialist who has first-hand experience of stuttering. He highlights the power of a group approach:

> There is nothing we cannot accomplish together. Living with and learning to control stuttering can be very challenging; you know that. I wish adults had told me that we will learn to control my stuttering together. Sometimes, adults felt sorry for me. Sometimes they spoke for me. A few clinicians even gave up on me; they didn't think I could control my stuttering. They were wrong. Sometimes adults can be wrong. I have learned that even the heaviest load (and stuttering can be a heavy load) seems lighter when it is shared. The load is best managed when working with clinicians and parents or guardians who understand stuttering and who are willing to work together. In the western part of the USA, there are big, very tall trees called Sequoias. Because the trees are so tall, people think their roots are very

deep. Actually, they are not. The trees stand strong and tall because they grow near each other and their roots overlap and grow together. Separately, the trees would fall; together they are strong. People facing big challenges such as stuttering are like that too; together we are stronger. We can accomplish anything together.

Yes, David, being together makes us stronger, and of all the triumphs which become possible when we work together, defeating isolation is undeniably the most beautiful.

I WISH I HAD KNOWN THAT I'D WRITE

THESE LINES ONE DAY

Walt Manning, a person who stutters and who has become a speech therapist once wrote:

> I would never want to give the impression that the path has been an easy one and without fear and failures. But, all things considered, it has been a grand adventure. Rather than my demon, I have come to regard my stuttering as a gift, something that has taken me to exciting places, provided me with opportunities for growth, and allowed me to meet wonderful people that I would never have met otherwise. Over the years I've heard other people who stutter say the same thing, and I know they mean it.

I can confirm what he says: I am living a wonderful adventure! When I posted that first article on my blog on 18 May 2009, I didn't think that it would change my life as radically as it has. That it would lead to writing more than 160 articles, and translating and publishing two American books. I have been invited to talk in public about my experience of stuttering. I have participated in radio programs, and have been interviewed by a journalist with a camera stuck in front of my nose. I have been invited all over France, and to Switzerland, Belgium and even Canada. There have been hundreds of encounters. And I have had the opportunity to link with other people who stutter from all over the world. And some of those people have come to mean a lot to me.

After having taken a great deal from me, stuttering has given me a great deal back. In the end, I have managed to transform my difference into a positive experience which has had repercussions on all aspects of my family life, my social life and my professional life. The result is that I now have a completely different way of approaching life; with the certainty that everything is possible, each adventure begins with the first step, every door opened reveals a new horizon and the only limits are the ones we set ourselves.

And that reminds me of myself as little boy afraid of asking for Ajax. I would have liked him to know all that.

I hope that you too will have delightful encounters and make great discoveries. That the days and years to come will be marked by the urge to try new things, the courage to get going, the strength to persevere and the joy of letting yourself go!

Yes, let's get going. Adventure is just round the corner!

Thanks

Thanks to Olivier, Alexandre, Daniel, François, Marie-Claude, Joseph, Margaret, John, Sarah, Lee, Morgane, Malcolm, John, Gary, Robert, Jack, Bérenger, Bill, Peter, Gerald, Tim, Harold, John, Patricia, Laure, Gilles, Jim, Lieven, Tom, Joe, Ryme, Fred, Nina, Silvano, David, Alan, Catherine, Hal, Mark, Clément, René, Charles, Lon, Walt, Anna, Pam, Amy, Patrick, Joe, Geneviève, Russ, Keith, Mohammed, Anne-Fleur, Betty and all those who have shared their experiences of people who stutter and therapists.

Your stories have been essential. I hope that this book will contribute to the spread of your precious words which would otherwise disappear too quickly into the limbo of social media.

Thanks to Steve (assisted by Veronica) for his translation and his always pertinent suggestions.

Thanks to Alan for rereading and encouragement, and for his wonderful and kind preface.

Thanks to Denis for his help for the cover design.

And thanks to that special person, she who saw beyond my stuttering, who was the first to guess what would help and who had the patience and intelligence to let me discover it for myself.

Resources

Associations

The Stuttering Foundation
www.stutteringhelp.org

National Stuttering Association
www.westutter.org

The British Stammering Association
www.stammering.org

Canadian Stuttering Association
www.stutter.ca

The Indian Stammering Association
indiastammering.com

Australian Speak Easy Association
www.speakeasy.org.au

Blogs

Mastering blocking and stuttering
masteringstuttering.com

Stuttering Jack
stutteringjack.com

Make room for the stuttering
stutterrockstar.com

Stuttering is cool
stutteringiscool.com

Made in the USA
Middletown, DE
17 March 2021